PLAISIRS

D' AMOUR

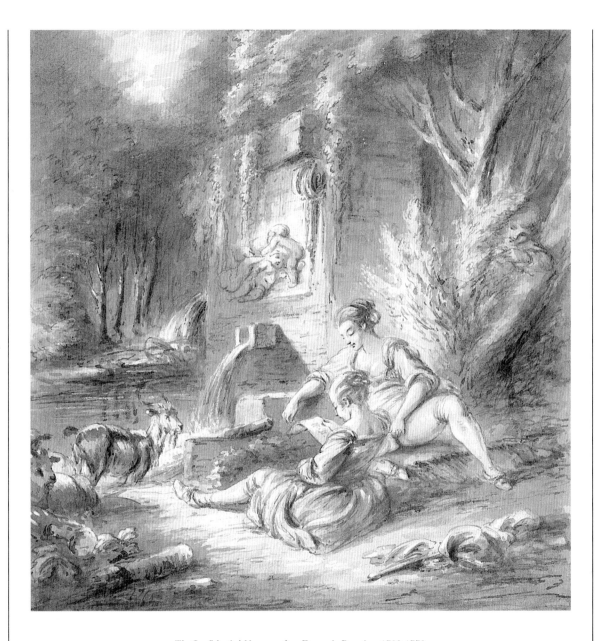

The Confidential Message, after François Boucher 1703-1770
The editors would like to express their gratitude to the Museum of Erotic Art, Hamburg, who generously permitted this drawing and more than thirty other items from their magnificent collection to be included in this book.

PLAISIRS

D'AMOUR

An erotic guide to
the senses

Elizabeth Nash

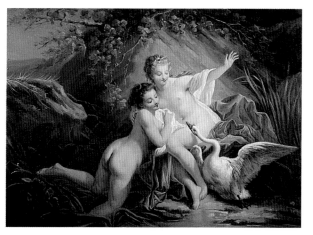

HarperSanFrancisco
A Division of HarperCollins*Publishers*

Plaisirs d'Amour: *An Erotic Guide to the Senses.*
Copyright (c) 1995 by CQ Editions. All rights reserved. Printed in Hong Kong.
No part of this book may be used
or reproduced in any manner whatsoever without written
permission except in the case of brief quotations embodied
in critical articles and reviews. For information, address
HarperCollins *Publishers*, 10 East 53rd Street, New York,
NY 10022.
Published in the United Kingdom by Pavilion Books Limited

FIRST EDITION

Library of Congress Cataloging-in-Publication Data
Nash, Elizabeth.
Plaisirs d'Amour: *An Erotic Guide to the senses*/Elizabeth Nash.
-- 1st ed.
p. cm.

ISBN 0-06-251149-1 (pbk. : acid-free paper)
1. Erotica. 2. Erotic art. 3. Erotic literature. I. Title.
HQ460.N37 1995
306. 7--dc20   94-23173
CIP
95 96 97 98 99 PAV 10 9 8 7 6 5 4 3 2 1

CONTENTS

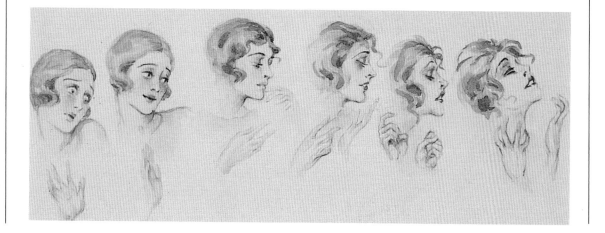

ACKNOWLEDGMENTS

Illustrations: *'Adam and Eve'* by Tamara de Lempicka is reproduced by kind permission of Kizette de Lempicka Foxhall and the Estate of Tamara de Lempicka. Fine Art Photographic Library of London provided more than fifty items from their unique archive of nineteenth-century British and European paintings. Egon Schiele's *'Legender weiblicher Akt mit gespreizten Beinen'* courtesy of the Graphische Sammlung Albertina, Vienna. Gustav Klimt's *'Adam and Eva'*; *'Goldfische'* and *'The Friends'* courtesy of Galerie Welz, Salzburg.

Two photographs of Rodin's *'Danaide'* taken by Bruno Jarret © ADAGP, Paris, and DACS London, and reproduced with permission of the Musée Rodin, Paris.
Two paintings by Julio Romero de Torres, *'Naranjas y Lìmones'* and *'La chiquita piconera'* by kind permission of the Museo Julio Romero de Torres, Cordoba.

The Erotic Art Museum in Hamburg provided more than thirty items from their extensive collection. The balance of the illustrations are from The Klinger Collection and Il Collezionista.
Text: Indra Sinha made new translations of Sanskrit poetry especially for this book. Elisabeth Ingles kindly provided the musicology for the section on Hearing.

While every effort has been made to trace all copyright holders this has proved difficult in some cases. The editors ask any copyright holders not mentioned to accept their apologies and to contact the publishers so that a proper credit can be made when the book reprints.

PAGE 3: *Nymphs and a Swan*, Jean Baptiste Huet 1745-1811.
PAGE 5: Watercolour by an unknown artist, circa 1930.
PAGE 7: *Sleeping Beauty*, Thomas Ralph Spence, 1855-1918.
PAGE 8: Drawing by H. Gerbault, circa 1890.

PREFACE

This is a book about erotic enjoyment, a celebration of the human senses. It is written – pleasurably – from the perspective of middle age, life's probable half-way point when the first cup has been drained enthusiastically and we hope to finish a second. If this essay encourages some of its readers to drink more deeply, then it has achieved its aim.

> They are not long, the days of wine and roses:
> Out of a misty dream
> Our path emerges for a while, then closes
> Within a dream

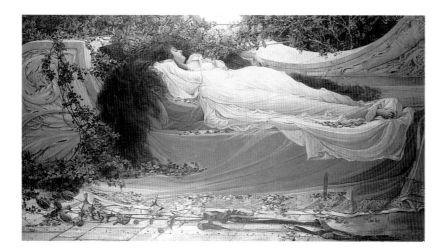

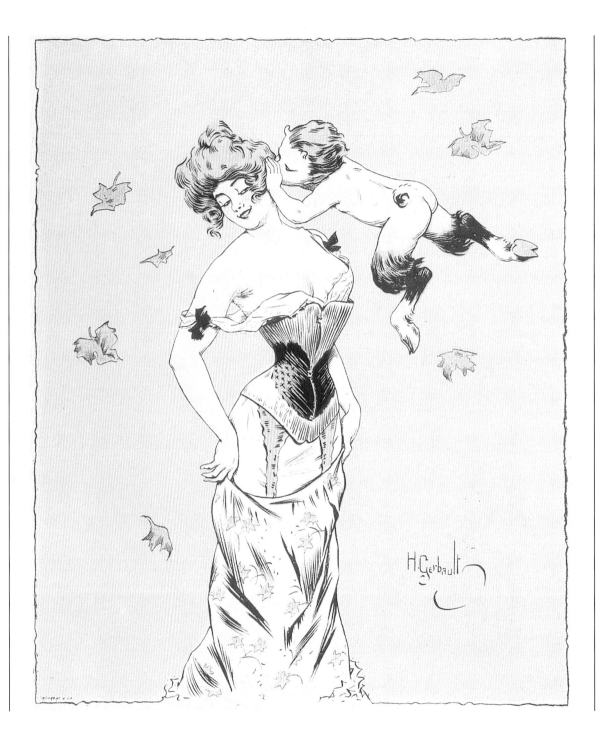

INTRODUCTION

Every book is a journey. For the writer it is a solitary business, re-visiting half-forgotten places and familiar landscapes in reflective mood. For the reader, a book is one of those journeys where – like it or not – every traveller is accompanied by a guide, the writer. Guides, as we all know, tend to follow their own agenda and seldom show us the things we would like to see. In this book we will try very hard to break with that convention. Unlike the guides in Pompeii or at Khajuraho, who traditionally need extra payment to show you the most sexually explicit items, we will withhold nothing. This is, after all, a book for adults about eroticism and the senses: even vulgar illustrations of sexuality have their place alongside sublime works of art and can sometimes tell us more. The commentary also includes quotations from a wide diversity of authors including the disreputable (and remarkably prolific) 'anonymous' – but what would travel be without colourful companions?

Sex is the only human activity which excites and engages all the senses: that is why it is so pleasurable, just as Nature intended it should be. (Nature in her generosity also compensates those who do not have a particular faculty by increasing the power of the senses that remain to a degree hard to imagine.) The fact that sex keeps our entire sensory quintet busy creates certain problems for the writer. What is the best way to approach the subject? An erotic consumers' guide in which a comprehensive list of sexual topics was analysed in terms of the five senses would at least take account of our complicated sensual response to sex. For example:

<small>CUNNILINGUS</small>

For the Giver: Vision and Touch – low score

                    Taste and Smell – high score

                    Hearing – muffled

For the Receiver: Touch – highest possible score

                    Other senses – Who cares?

But where are all the associations and cultural subtleties which make human sexuality so delightful and so much more than the merely animal? If we feel the need to append an essay to each entry surely it would be better to choose a more sympathetic structure from the outset?

The alternative approach – which we have chosen – is to examine each sense in turn: Sight, Taste, Smell, Hearing and Touch. This allows for the inclusion of a wide variety of material which would otherwise be omitted. It is a more interesting approach, but not without its problems. Where do you put Cunnilingus, in Touch? No, the answer is Taste. Male and female orality can then be dealt with together (the common feature being the mouth which contains the organs of taste) and more satisfactorily. Similar 'logic' will place baths and bathroom topics in the section concerned with Smell, but bathing and water under Touch. The fact is that the senses, like Nature, abhor straight lines or confinement of any kind and some erotic themes will be dealt with in unexpected places or in more than one section.

Among the host of illustrations in this book, jostling one another for aesthetic or erotic appeal, there is a recurring image: Adam and Eve. This could have been accidental – they are one of the most popular icons in Western art, being conveniently nude yet respectable – but it is not. Adam and Eve are a constant reminder of our inheritance: the differences between the sexes, the importance of a mutually supportive relationship, the possibility of love. The archetypal man and woman lost paradise and immortality, but found their humanity. A return to the infantile pleasures of the Garden of Eden can hardly compare with the love a sensual man and woman can enjoy.

We began this introduction with an imaginative journey and end it with a suggestion for a real one. Go and see Jan Van Eyck's great altar-piece in Sint-Baafskathedral in Gent. Go, because to actually see a great work of art is a visceral, sensual experience no book or print can ever give you. There, from their panels on opposite sides of the glorious altar-piece with its mystical message of Christian redemption, they look at each other as they have for more than five centuries. He is an unidealized naked man, self-aware, his eyes hot with who knows what thoughts. She dreams rather, and makes little attempt to conceal the pubic hair beneath her rounded Gothic belly. They are truthful in a way that defies description this Adam and Eve, they are us.

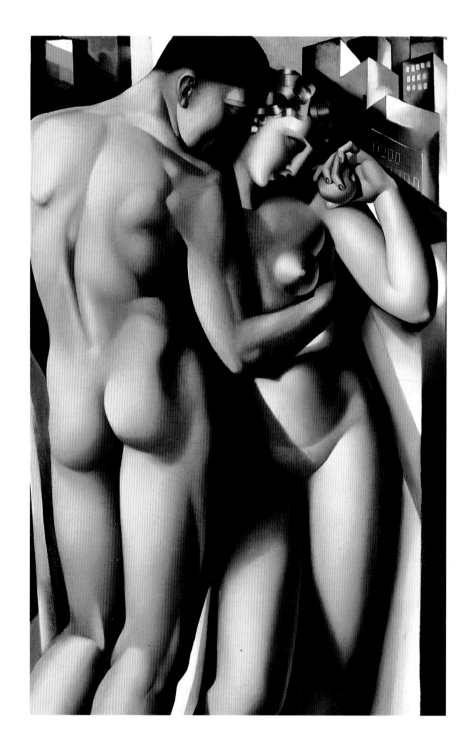

S I G H T

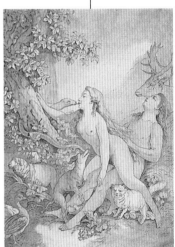

And when the woman saw that the tree was good for food, and that it was pleasant to the eyes, and a tree to be desired to make one wise, she took of the fruit thereof, and did eat, and gave also unto her husband with her; and he did eat. And the eyes of them both were opened, and they knew that they were naked...

THE BOOK OF GENESIS

Of all the gifts we have received, of all our five senses, sight is perhaps the most precious. As the first among equals, sight imposes order in the chaotic world of the senses. Sight also has direct access to the higher functions of the human brain and holds the key to the hidden world of the unconscious. The very fact that this thought can be expressed in this way – using the metaphor of a key – is because the sense of sight has allowed us to develop the powerful language of symbolism.

OPPOSITE PAGE: *Adam and Eve*, Tamara de Lempicka, 1898-1980
ABOVE: *The Garden of Eden*, artist unknown

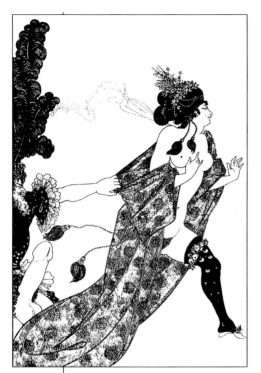

In the mythologies of many peoples the sun is associated with the eye. The logic is impeccable: as an organ the eye is our response to the light which shines from the first of all the gods. The coloured part of the eye, the iris, takes its name from the nymph associated with the rainbow. The pupil, more prosaically, is from the Latin 'pupilla' meaning doll because we see a tiny doll-like reflection of ourselves when we look into the dark centre of the eye. It comes as no surprise that Captain Hook and Long John Silver were not among the Caribbean's more successful pirates: binocular vision is important if predators are to judge speed and distance efficiently.

Eyes are not only the windows through which we see beauty, they are themselves beautiful:

'She walks in beauty, like the night
Of cloudless climes and starry skies;
And all that's best of dark and bright
Meet in her aspect and her eyes.'

Lord Byron (1788-1824)

The importance of eyes in sexual attraction can hardly be exaggerated. We seek out the eyes of someone to whom we are initially attracted with the ruthless perseverance of an inquisitor. Are their eyes also attractive? What is the true personality behind them? Is there any reciprocal interest or feeling? What is the nature and extent of that interest? This aspect of human behaviour, which we all practise however light-heartedly, has given rise to a wealth of courtship language. We talk of 'giving someone the eye' and sing that we 'only have eyes for you.' Someone can be 'the apple' of our eye, which is an old term for the pupil and – if we are lucky – we may receive 'the glad eye.' There is no doubt that a good deal of information can be exchanged 'eye to eye' but, as in all means of communication, disastrous misunderstandings can also occur. 'Bedroom eyes' should be put on with rather more prior consideration than bedroom slippers.

RIGHT: *A Venetian Beauty*, Eugene de Blaas, 1843-1931
OPPOSITE PAGE: *Cinesias entreating Myrrhina to Coition* (from Lysistrata), Aubrey Beardsley, 1872-1898

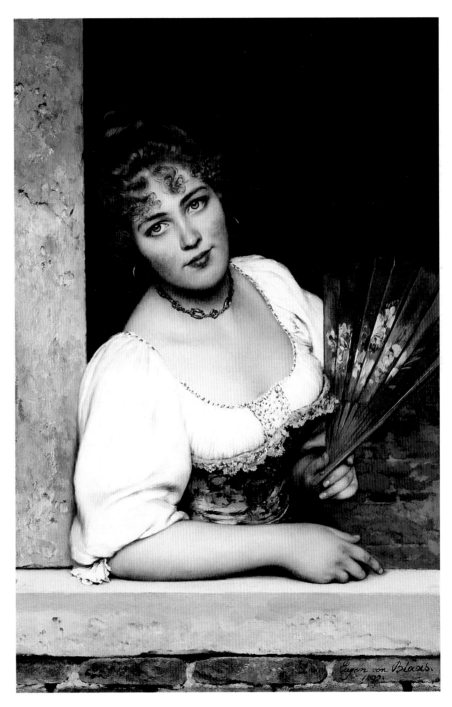

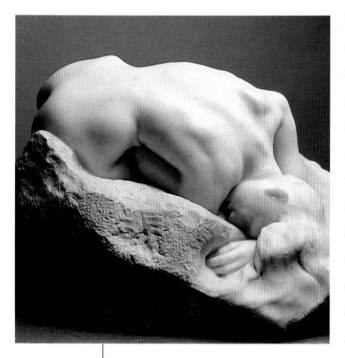

The technology of war and aggression can often be turned to better use: the bronze smelting and casting techniques of the ancient world, developed first for swords and arrowheads, made possible the glories of Classical Greek sculpture. Our eyes – the essential equipment of aggressive hunter-gatherers, organs in which evolution has concentrated nearly three-quarters of the body's sensory receptors – open on to a world our primitive ancestors could not have dreamed of. Yet it is to them that we owe the wonder of sight. Because our ancestors watched antelopes in order to understand better how to kill them, we can enjoy the drama and excitement of movement.

Because the hunter needs to know instantaneously which stone to reach for to defend himself or to kill his prey, we can appreciate the sensual planes and contours of sculpture. Later it was that same hunter, painting his prey on a cave wall in simple pigments for totemic reasons, who gave us the beginning of art. We should not forget pigment. Our eyes also decode the secrets of the spectrum for us, so that all the colours in the world burst upon our senses.

From the earliest times we have borrowed from the infinitely varied sex life of plants to enhance and dramatize our own. Perfume will be dealt with elsewhere, but colour has an equally important role to play in eroticism. Until comparatively recently we needed to borrow substances from nature to produce pigments. Today we can produce dyes chemically, but our enjoyment and understanding of colour is inextricably bound up with nature, and with flowers in particular.

The age-old gift of flowers – simple and picked in the wild or from a garden, or elaborate and shop-bought – is still the best present lovers can exchange. Children, and adults, will always pluck petals from flowers to divine if someone 'loves them', or 'loves them not'. Every town and city in the Western world has its flower shops. Of course flowers mark sad occasions as well as joyful ones, but whenever we need to express emotions that are beyond words, we say it with flowers.

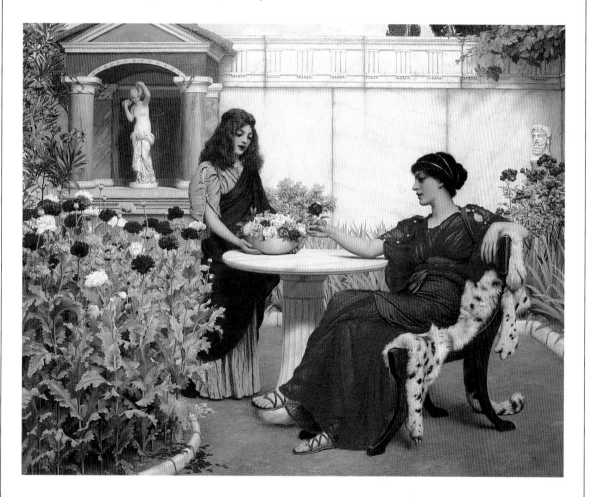

OPPOSITE PAGE: *La Danaide,* Auguste Rodin, 1840-1917
ABOVE: *Choosing,* John William Godward, 186l-1922

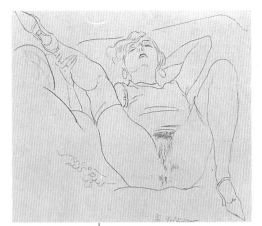

Symbolism is intimately connected with the power of sight and visual memory; as are its literary offspring metaphor (Greek meta, 'across'; phor-a, 'carrying') and simile (Latin similis, 'like'). One thing may represent another thing either by convention or because of some deep unconscious resonance beyond words. The language of flowers has its conventional and polite form in which anemone means refusal, foxglove insincerity, gardenia secret love and so on. Most of this language is concerned with courtship.

Lady Mary Wortley Montagu (1690-1762), elaborating on the meanings ascribed to flowers since ancient times, declared that it was possible to 'send letters of passion…without even inking your fingers.' Much of this has its origins in Classical mythology, where Aphrodite's grief made anemones spring from the blood of dead Adonis, and poor Clytie was turned into a sunflower, doomed for eternity to turn her head and watch her beloved Apollo, the sun god, cross the heavens each day.

There is another language of flowers. The rose represents the Love goddess in most traditions. It is an unmistakable symbol: the colour of a traditional rose and its unfolding petals making it the archetypal female emblem. Orchids are rather less subtle, their hothouses like steamy bordellos with lines of brazen inmates lewdly exposing themselves. Frank Harris employs a flower simile to describe the sex of the voracious Mrs Mayhew in *My Life and Loves* (1925), calling the lips 'madder-brown' although the rest of the description owes more to an orchid catalogue: 'her clitoris was much more than the average button: it stuck out fully half an inch and the inner lips of her vulva hung down a little below the outer lips…'

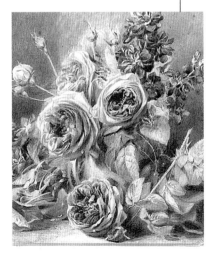

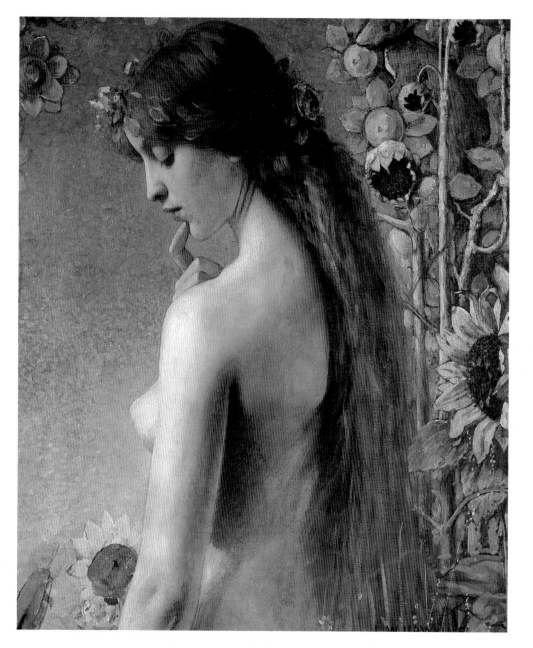

ABOVE: *Clytie*, Louise Weldon Hawkins, died 1910
OPPOSITE PAGE, TOP: Drawing by Rudolf Schlichter, 1890-1955
OPPOSITE PAGE, BOTTOM: *Roses*, Mary Margetts, died 1886

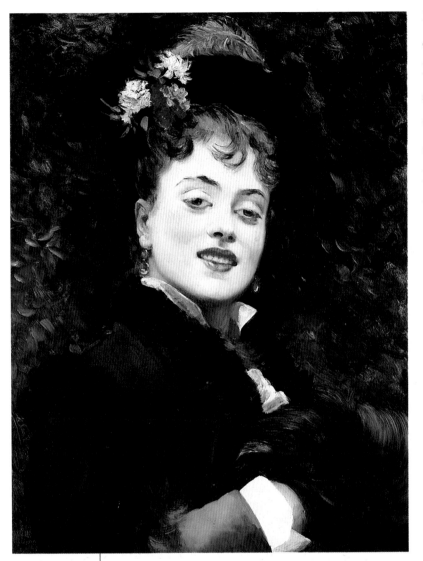

Frank Harris (1855-1931) was, on his own admission, not in love with Lorna Mayhew and that coloured (literally) all of his descriptions of her. Compare these lines from the poet Jayadeva's *Gitagovindam*, a lyrical account of the lovemaking of Krishna and Radha written in the twelfth century AD:

> Lady with lotus eyes,
> Reclining on your bed of leaves,
> Untie your belt,
> Let fall your petticoat,
> And part your pretty thighs
> That he who loves you may
>   delight
> In gazing on your hidden jewel.

It is important to see our sexual organs as things of beauty, and not only because 'Love looks not with the eyes but with the mind.' A journalist, herself beautiful, once complained that she could never understand why men used the word 'cunt' as the ultimate expression of contempt when it was the name for the most beautiful part of a woman. There is no excuse, but perhaps the reason is the power in the word, the same impulse that drives us to blaspheme.

Colour as well as shape, is important if we are to understand that our sex organs can be looked at aesthetically and that pudenda (Latin pudere, 'to be ashamed') is a word to be left unused in the dictionary. John Cleland (1709-1789) in his magnificent erotic novel *Fanny Hill*, describes both men and women beautifully, although perhaps with a little too much vermilion on his palette. Fanny spies upon Polly: 'Her thighs were spread out to their utmost extension, and discovered between them the mark of her sex, the red-centred cleft of flesh, whose lips, vermilioning inwards, expressed a small ruby line in sweet miniature...' Fanny Hill's description of her lover Charles is no less charming:

'I, struggling faintly, could not help feeling what I could not grasp, a column of the whitest ivory, beautifully streak'd with blue veins, and carrying, fully uncapt, a head of the liveliest vermilion; no horn could be harder and stiffer; yet no velvet more smooth or delicious to the touch.'

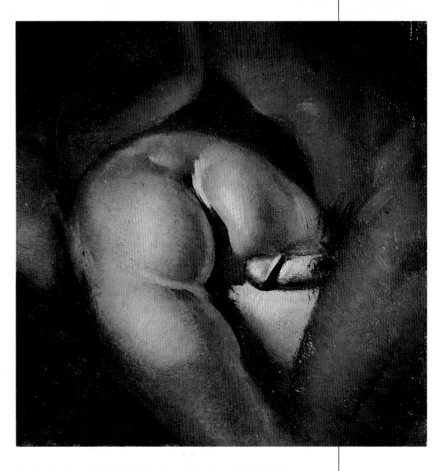

Our aesthetic appreciation of colour, and our ability to see or imagine one thing as another, are a powerful force in sexual attraction. What are the moistly parted red lips of Garreta's model but the emblem, and sisters, of her other lips?

OPPOSITE PAGE: *Portrait of a young lady,* Raimundo de Madrazo y Garreta, 1841-1920
ABOVE: Oil painting by an unknown Italian master

I can love both fair and brown,

Her whom abundance melts, and her whom want

   betrays,

Her who loves loneness best, and her whom masks

   and plays,

Her whom the country form'd, and whom the

   town,

Her who believes, and her who tries,

Her who still weeps with spongy eyes,

And her who is a dry cork, and never cries;

I can love her, and her, and you and you,

I can love any, so she be not true.

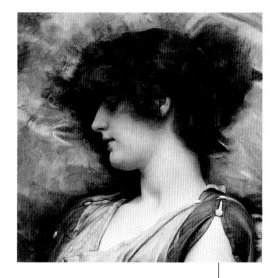

from *The Indifferent*, John Donne (1571-1631)

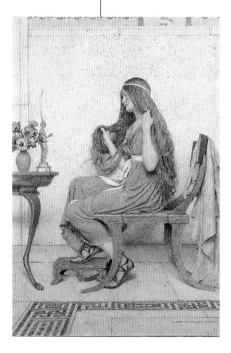

The colour of hair is often the first thing we seize upon to describe an individual. This is due in part to our strong unconscious response to colour. But hair coloration is also a useful shorthand since it very often implies other associated colour values; the alabaster-white skin of the redhead, the olive skin that often goes with black hair, and so on. Obviously this is an unreliable code and dangerous in the wrong hands. We are so attuned to colour that we can, and do, seize upon it to distinguish one from another as if it had some relevance beyond aesthetics. And even with aesthetics we should remember that beauty, in the end, is personal and subjective. The vitriol Shakespeare throws at the 'dark lady' in *Sonnet 130* is an example of the values colour should not be credited with:

My mistres eyes are nothing like the Sunne,

Currall is farre more red, than her lips red,

If snow be white, why then her brests are dun:

If haires be wiers, black wiers grow on her head:

I have seene Roses damaskt, red and white,

But no such Roses see I in her cheekes...

A happier comment on hair coloration is to be found in the pastiche novel *Passion's Apprentice:* 'Marie-Louise had flowing auburn hair and the milky skin which often accompanies that colouring... he was behind her, lifting the soft weight of her breasts with one hand, and exploring between her legs with the other. He tore off his clothes and dropped to his knees behind her. She bent her legs a little and pushed out her buttocks so that he could lick her. Her body perfume was intense, the taste of her scarlet sex like ripe fruit that has burst open'.

OPPOSITE PAGE BOTTOM: *The Looking Glass,* George Lawrence Bulleid, 1858-1933

OPPOSITE PAGE TOP: *Faraway Thoughts,* John William Godward, 1861-1922

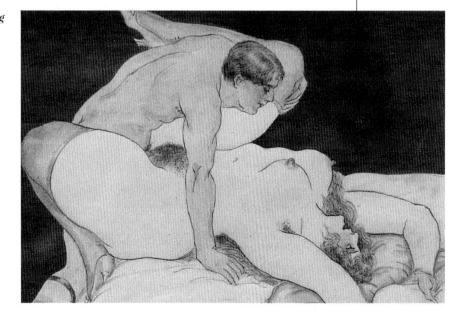

RIGHT: *Redhead,* unknown Czech artist, circa 1900

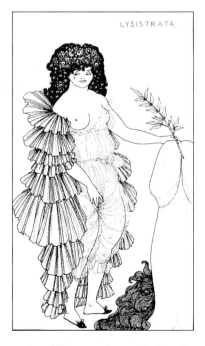

When Nature is pleased with a shape she tends to stay with it, reproducing that form in surprisingly different circumstances . It is safer, though, to regard the similarities between erect penises and cucumbers, as a joke rather than an identical response to gravity and friction. Many fruit forms are strongly suggestive of the penis, and it is not unknown for these similarities to go beyond visual enjoyment. Sir Richard Burton (1821-1890) recorded that the women of the harem were never allowed the long white radishes popular in the East 'unless they first be sliced.' No doubt the eunuchs who attended them carried out this culinary task with assiduity, having themselves experienced the unkindest cut of all.

The Romans often used vegetable metaphors to describe the penis, including thysus (stalk) arbor (tree) and radix (root). The testicles completed the erotic salad with fabae (beans) and mala (apples). Their ithyphallic god Priapus was the custodian of horticulture; his statue was erected (literally) in fields and orchards throughout the Empire.

Our culture tends to prefer mechanical (tool) or even military (weapon) allusions. The Hindu god Shiva, whose sacred emblem is the penis (lingam), is Lord of both Creation and Destruction. Ironically, the phallic sword which appears in many depictions of Shiva has been superseded in our times by even more penile weapons of destruction: guns, bullets, shells and the ballistic missile.

This aggressive paraphernalia is, of course, all about insecurity. The much symbolised

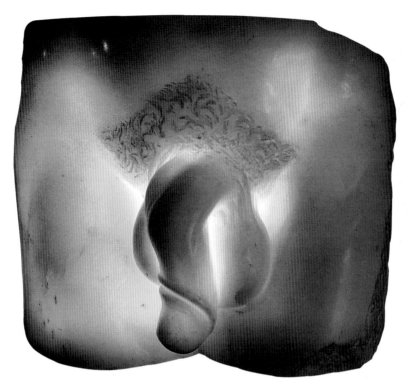

penis – with its bombastic and not always perfect transitions – can itself be regarded as a symbol of the dual nature of the male: both strong and vulnerable. Humour is the best antidote to phallic self-importance. We all know the identity of the real tempter in the Garden of Eden, and the penile snake features in many legends. The caricature of Laocoon fighting the sea serpents is an unorthodox depiction although it was his penis that got him into trouble in the first place.

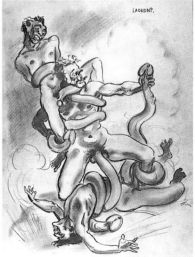

OPPOSITE PAGE, TOP: *The Worship of Priapus,* neo-classical, artist unknown
OPPOSITE PAGE, BOTTOM: *Lysistrata,* Aubrey Beardsley
TOP: *The Penis,* alabaster, nineteenth century, artist unknown
RIGHT: *Laocoon,* anonymous

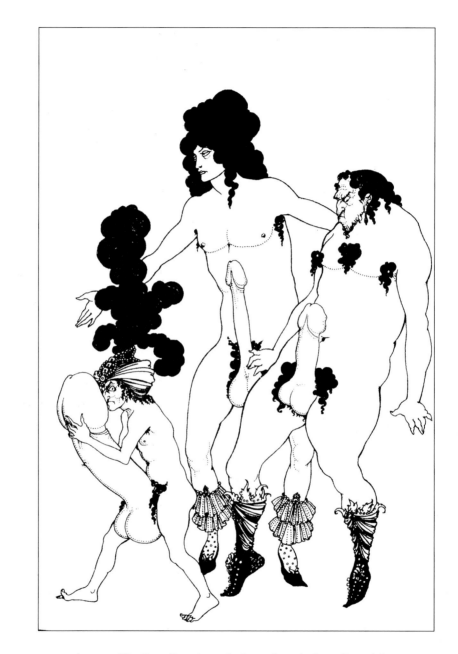

ABOVE: *The Lacadaemonian Ambassadors,* Aubrey Beardsley
OPPOSITE PAGE, TOP: *High Jinks,* anonymous, circa 1890
OPPOSITE PAGE, BOTTOM: Shunga woodblock print, eighteenth century

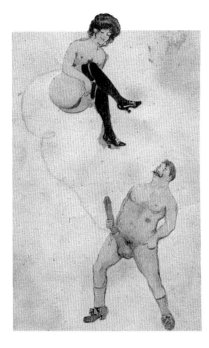

The artists who produced shunga, the erotic prints of Japan, were not concerned with realism. The gigantic penises which characterize their incandescent erotica are the artistic equivalent of fireworks – an artificial creation intended to shock and amaze.

Aubrey Beardsley's 'Lacadaemonian Ambassadors' from the Lysistrata series was drawn with the same intention; he was much influenced by shunga and collected it. This essentially humorous approach to sex – and penile size in particular – is both enabling and instructive, since an obsessive concern with size (as with 'beauty' or 'slimness') is corrosive. A big penis makes a good show, but humour helps us put it in its place (as it were).

Fanny Hill has the last word on the subject: 'Curious then, and eager to unfold so alarming a mystery, playing, as it were, with his buttons which were bursting ripe from the active force within, those of his waistband and fore-flap flew open at a touch, when out it started; and now, disengag'd from the shirt, I saw, with wonder and surprise, what? Not the plaything of a boy, not the weapon of a man, but a maypole of so enormous a standard, that had proportions been observ'd, it must have belonged to a young giant!'

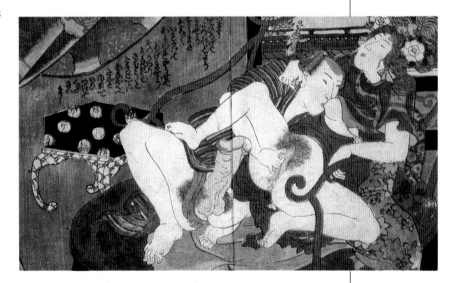

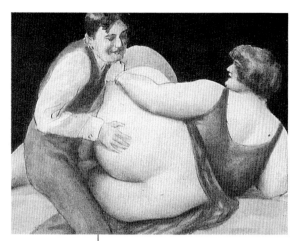

Our eye, itself round, delights in round forms. The same inbuilt sense which 'knows' that angular shapes and things which stick up are 'male', recognizes round forms as 'female'. We are of course talking of buttocks and breasts. Nature likes her joke however, and to the surprise of many men their bottoms are of erotic interest to women, or they can be. This needs some qualification. While women favour the hard and compact 'apple' behind, men hunger for shapes best described in terms of pears, peaches and even melons. There are differences too of degree. The erotic frisson which the sight of a pert male behind may afford a woman is not to be compared to the abiding passion which her derrière can kindle in him. The poet Paul Verlaine (1844-1896) – who knew and loved the bottoms of both men and women – wrote a eulogy to 'the glory of a woman's arse':

> Cul féminin, vainqueur serein du cul viril,
> Fût-il éphébéen, et fût-il puéril,
> Cul féminin, cul sur tous culs, los,
>   culte et gloire!

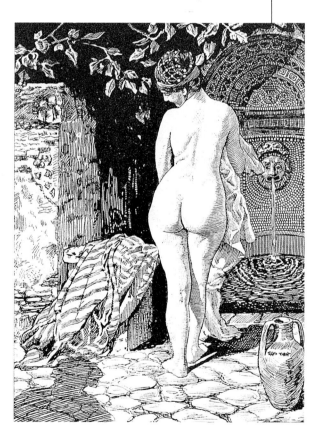

The inhabitants of ancient Syracuse dedicated a temple to the love goddess where she was worshipped in her incarnation as Venus Callipygos or 'Venus of the beautiful buttocks.'

The seventeenth-century Spanish noblewoman Aloysia Sigea recalls a different kind of worship:

'When he saw my buttocks, whiter than ivory and snow, 'How beautiful you are!' he cried, 'But raise yourself on your knees, and bend your head down.' I bowed my head and bosom, and lifted my buttocks. He thrust his swift-moving and fiery dart deep in my vagina and took one of my nipples in either hand. Then he began to work in and out, and soon sent a sweet rivulet into the shrine of Venus. I also felt unspeakable delight and nearly fainted with lust.'

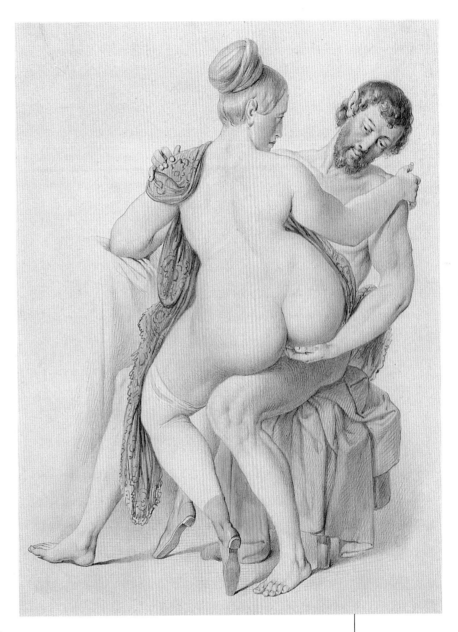

RIGHT: *Lovers*, Johann Nepomuk Geiger, 1805-1880

OPPOSITE PAGE, TOP: Untitled watercolour by an anonymous Czech artist
OPPOSITE PAGE, BOTTOM: An illustration from Erotici, Adolfo Magrini

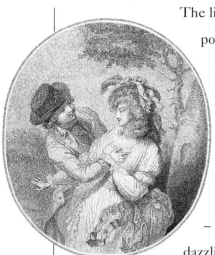

The link between breasts and buttocks is more than aesthetic, and possibly more than accidental. Desmond Morris proposed the fascinating theory that as our ancestors became more upright, the breasts of the female enlarged to replace buttocks as the primary sexual focus for the male. Verlaine anticipated the idea in his brilliant poem *Partie carrée* which compares breasts and buttocks. It was here he coined the unforgettable phrase 'Buttocks, big sisters of the breasts.' Comparison is invidious – as all sisters know – but the extraordinary variety of shape, colour and movement is so dazzling that it seems to support the idea that breasts are a cunning erotic confection. The fact that the nipples change shape and colour with sexual excitement is Nature's final virtuoso flourish.

Fanny Hill had a good eye for breasts: 'This girl could not be above eighteen: her face regular and sweet-featur'd, her shape exquisite; nor could I help envying her two ripe enchanting breasts, finely plump'd out in flesh, but withal so round, so firm, that they sustain'd themselves, in scorn of any stay: then their nipples, pointing different ways, mark'd their pleasing separation...'

Size in breasts is less important to the male than might be supposed: lovers in search of amplitude can always resort to big sisters. 'Champagne glass' breasts where the nipples are often large in proportion are just as exciting in their way as Rabelaisian goblets.

Just as males (heterosexual males at least) tend to forget that men have buttocks, so women tend to forget that men have nipples. They are not as large or as beautiful as female nipples, but they are highly erogenous for all that. Male nipples did not escape Fanny Hill's notice: 'The platform of his snow-white bosom, that was laid out in a manly proportion, presented on the vermilion summit of each pap, the idea of a rose about to bloom.'

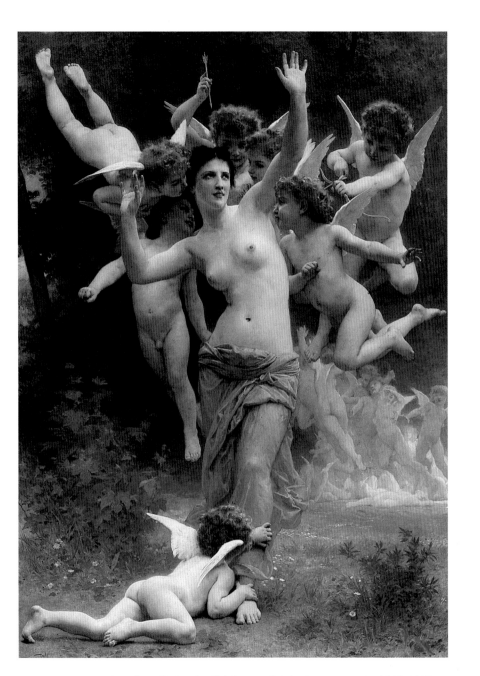

ABOVE: *Invading Cupid's Realm*, William Adolphe Bouguereau, 1825-1905
OPPOSITE PAGE: Eighteenth-century engraving, artist unknown

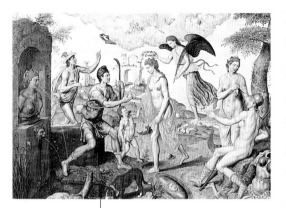

Ideals of physical beauty change and what is beautiful to one is not to another. When Faust made his bargain with Mephistopheles for one night with Helen of Troy he was not only risking his immortal soul, he was risking disappointment: ideals of beauty change in two millennia. We know the ancient Greek ideal for the female body from their sculpture. The female nude always conformed to an exact proportion in which the distance between the nipples equals both the distance from below the breasts to the navel, and the distance from the navel to the sex: the Classical Nude. The Faust legend is medieval in origin and by then the so-called Gothic Nude – with an elongated, pear-like belly and small breasts – epitomized female beauty. But Dr Faustus was not disappointed:

> 'Was this the face that launched a thousand ships
> And burnt the topless towers of Ilium?
> Sweet Helen, make me immortal with a kiss!'

Christopher Marlowe's evocative words are a little unfair to Helen who had less to do with causing the disastrous Trojan war than her impetuous lover Paris. Beauty was again the problem. The famous 'Judgement of Paris' showed an extraordinary lack of that very thing. Having first allowed himself to be appointed as judge, he was then foolish enough to make a pronouncement as to which of three goddesses (Aphrodite, Minerva and Hera) was the most beautiful. In choosing the goddess of Love, he naturally offended the goddess of War and the Queen of the gods, Hera. His reward from Aphrodite was to marry the most beautiful woman in the world, Helen. Unfortunately Helen was married to Menelaus who took it rather badly when the couple 'eloped' to Troy. And the rest is mythology. Morals are strikingly absent in the tales of Greek gods and heroes, but the moral here is that beauty is not an absolute: it knows no laws or rules, it is entirely subjective and personal. Each of us is an amalgam of parts, some beautiful, some not.

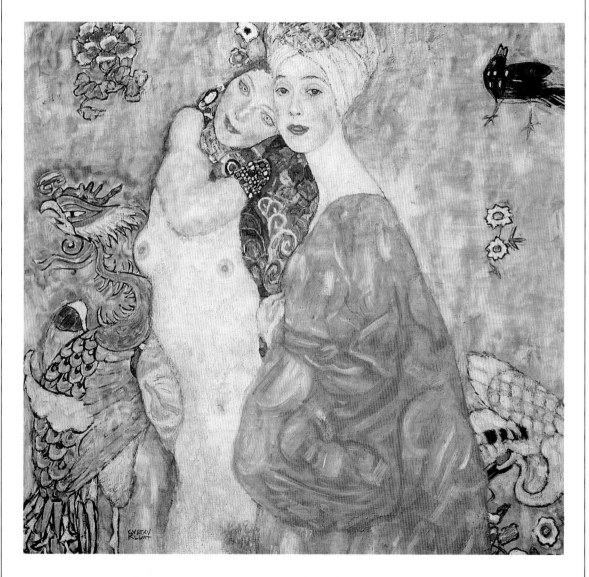

ABOVE: *Die Freundinnen,* Gustav Klimt, 1862-1918 (destroyed by fire in the Immendorf Palace)
OPPOSITE PAGE: *The Judgement of Paris,* Franco-Flemish School, sixteenth century, artist unknown

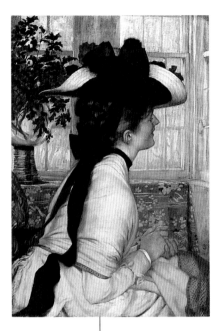

Human beings have always sought ways to enhance their appearance in order to make themselves more sexually attractive, often by exaggerating features which have erotic significance. The first of our natural attributes to receive attention was probably the hair (although the penis sheaths and extensions favoured by contemporary 'stone-age' peoples might suggest a rival focus of attention).

We are concerned here with the visual significance of hair, although of course it is also intimately associated with the senses of smell and touch. While flowers, ribbons and simple decoration are a way of enhancing the colour and interest of the hair, hats give height and importance. Elaborate, built-up hairstyles are another way of emphasizing the all-important head. Different coiffure can be designed to frame the face or to give the excitement of movement. During the High Victorian period it was possible to achieve all these objectives.

Although armpit hair is mainly concerned with scent it also interests and surprises the eye, particularly in an age when it is removed by many people. Pubic hair adds drama to the planes of thighs and belly, and by colour and change of texture draws eyes and attention to the delights below.

TOP: *Portrait of a Woman*, Jacques Joseph Tissot, 1836-1902
BOTTOM: *Lysistrata Haranguing the Athenian Women*, Aubrey Beardsley
OPPOSITE PAGE: *Queen for a Day*, Paul F. Poole, 1807-1879

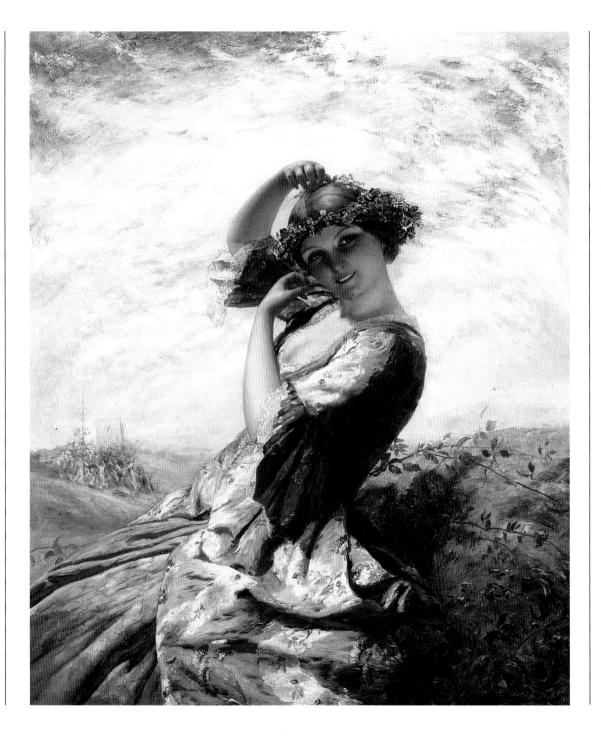

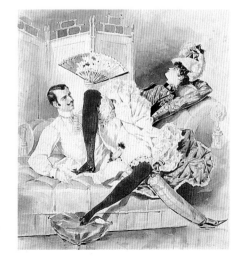

The practice of colouring and decorating the body, although it has ritualistic and magical origins, is concerned principally with sexual attraction in the developed world. Piercing is generally restricted to ears, although noses and nipples – and labia and penises for those with specialized sexual tastes – are becoming more common. Cutting is restricted to the foreskin, but although circumcised penises certainly look different circumcision is not generally regarded as a cosmetic adjustment. In sexual surveys some women with a marked preference for a circumcised penis (opinion is equally divided) have said that the frilly edge of the unretracted foreskin on a flaccid penis is somehow 'feminine'. Perhaps the origins of circumcision are cosmetic after all.

Jewellery gives light, colour and movement to the body. It also emphasizes features and creates an exciting new landscape by interrupting the eye as it moves across surfaces. We can learn a good deal about jewellery (and about eroticism) from the courtesans of India who made love naked – except for their elaborate jewellery. Because it implies the dressed state, and is a constant reminder of it, jewellery heightens the awareness of nudity and thus the erotic effect. Nature, as always, generously provides us with a treasure trove of minerals and organic substances which jewellers make into sensuous talismans.

The fan is an erotic accessory which became incredibly popular during the eighteenth century when a regular trade with the East was established. Apart from its very practical function, the decorated fan lent flashes of vivid colour to a lady's ensemble and distributed her personal perfume. In skilled

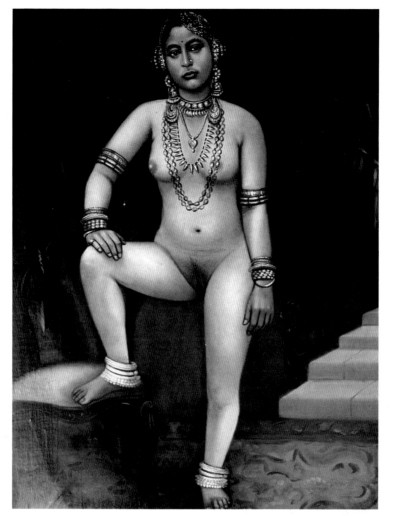

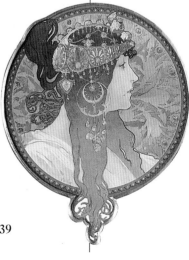

hands it was also capable of conveying amorous messages ranging from disdain to fluttering acquiescence.

ABOVE: *The Favourite,* late nineteenth century, India, artist unknown
OPPOSITE PAGE, TOP AND RIGHT: *The Blonde and the Brunette,* Alfons Mucha, 1860-1939
OPPOSITE PAGE, BOTTOM: Watercolour, Louis Morin, born 1851

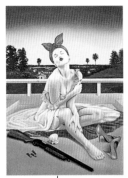

The human face, with its infinite repertoire of expressions conveying every nuance of emotion, is also susceptible to adjustment. Men, in the West at least, generally restrict these adjustments to removing or shaping facial hair, either to suit an image of themselves they are pleased with and wish to project, or for functional reasons. Ernest Hemingway (1899-1961) maintained that he shaved only when making love. (Hemingway had reason to be sensitive on tonsorial matters. Gertrude Stein in vindictive mood once described his writing as 'false hair on the chest.')

Makeup is the prerogative of women and is widely used. The apparent structure of the face can be altered by shaping and accentuating the eyebrows; by shading cheeks and covering reflective features like the nose and forehead. Blemishes can be masked, colour added and colour taken away. Eyes and lips can be defined or coloured, or both. None of this is new. We know from visual evidence that Egyptian women wore the most elaborate eye makeup as early as 3000 BC; the same was true in Minoan Crete, in fact all civilizations have used facial cosmetics to some degree.

Today in the West the type and colour of makeup used by women varies enormously. Some use muted pastels with minimal eye makeup, others accentuate eyes and paint lips in a way once used exclusively by streetwalkers to advertise the nature of their calling . The fact that prostitutes traditionally used heavy make-up is a clue to the original, largely unconscious purpose of the key features of makeup. The women of Ancient Egypt used chemicals to artificially enlarge their pupils, imitating the dilation which occurs with orgasm. Naturally this would have sent a strong subliminal message to men once the eye liner and colour had lured them into the centre of those bottomless pools. Rouge and its modern equivalents which colour cheeks convey a similar idea by copying orgasmic flushes. Knowing now the explicitly sexual function of facial makeup, we can let moistened and inviting carmine lips speak for themselves.

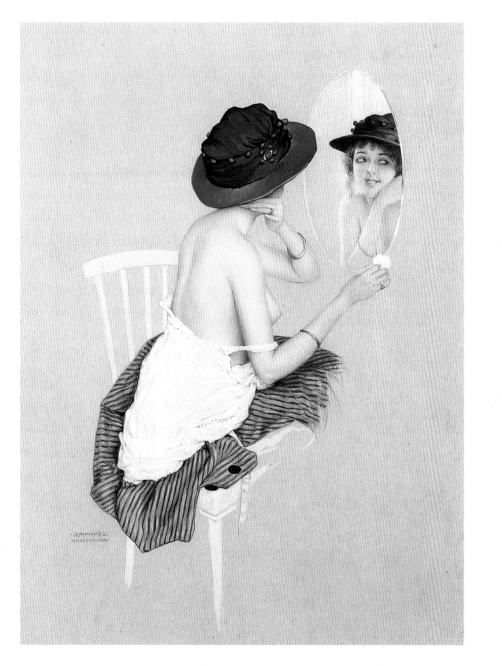

ABOVE: *The Blue Hat,* Raphael Kirchner, 1876-1917
OPPOSITE PAGE: *L.A. Promise,* Nikola Neubauer, contemporary

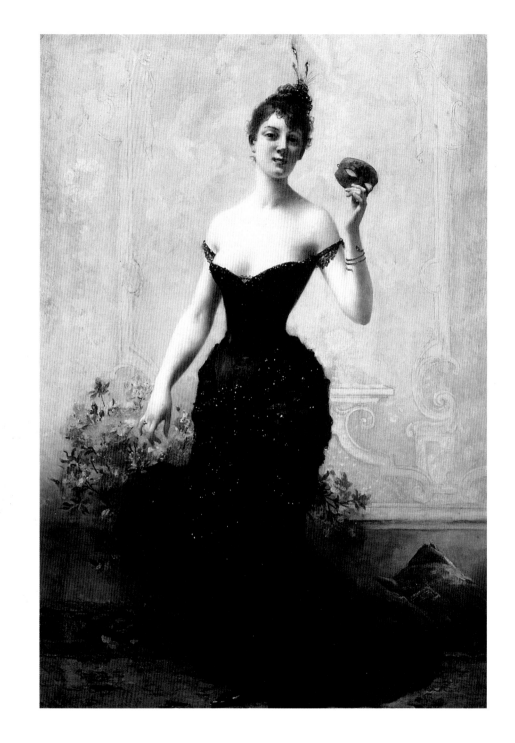

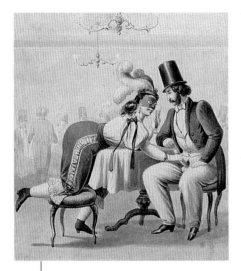

To look at the sun, for example during an eclipse, we make a small hole in a piece of card and study its projected image. The power of the sun is so great that we are blinded if we look directly at it. Some of the appeal of eye masks is that they function in much the same way. The power of the human face is so great that by partially covering it enough personality is projected to be interesting, while we are left to resolve any ambiguities by paying more attention to lips, body language and the voice. Total masks are more extreme because in wearing them we borrow a personality through which we must express our own wishes and desires. The Latin for mask is persona.

The other important feature of masks is that they lend anonymity, either real or feigned. People do things they would not normally do while concealed by masks: the executioner hides from God; Dick Turpin hides from the magistrates and the Lone Ranger hides from Tonto. The sinister aspect of masks needs to be mentioned but we are concerned here with pleasure and the enhancement of life. Masked balls, much favoured by Victorians, are tremendous fun. So is Carnival, and at least once everyone should go to Venice or one of the other great pre-Lent celebrations of life.

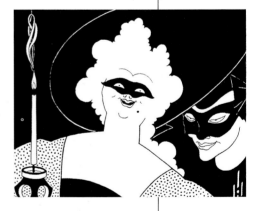

OPPOSITE PAGE: *Ready for the Masked Ball,* Jules Frederick Ballavoine, nineteenth century
TOP: Anonymous lithograph, Italy, nineteenth century
BOTTOM: Front cover image for The Yellow Book, April 1894, Aubrey Beardsley

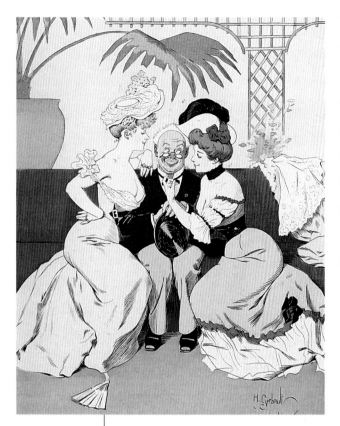

In the age of ready-made clothes it is easy to forget what a skilled tailor or dressmaker is actually doing – and why. The mating displays of birds parallel our own so closely that the language is full of ornithological metaphor: peacock, coxcomb, preening and so on. In a crueller age we even borrowed the feathers which the wretched creatures used in their sexual displays to enhance our own.

Colour in clothing is all-important, it is the first impression which beats upon our senses. Once we

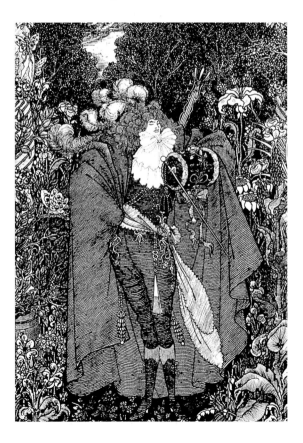

gathered feathers and leaves, now we print them on fabric along with other borrowings from Nature and geometric patterns of our own devising. Richly sensual coloured fabrics are not suitable for all purposes. Where the tailor is concerned with structure, solid plain colours are easier to manipulate.

Clothes designers have been so inventive, so remorseless in their search

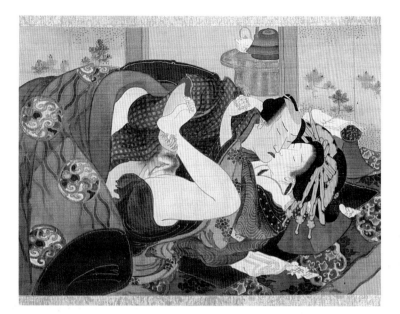

for sexual tricks, that we can only review a few of their manipulations. Men once accentuated their genitals with padded codpieces which ranged in size from very large to gigantic. The less satisfactory but more honest modern trend is to gather one's own assets in a sling-like pouch which makes as much of them as possible. The mini-skirt was a revelation in every sense, but actually less sexy than the Victorian 'waspie' corset and bustle which transformed a lady's derrière into a moving request to be mounted from the rear. Padded, angular shoulders which were once used to emphasize a secondary male sexual characteristic are now popular with women, as are trousers, in what amounts to a socially acceptable form of cross-dressing.

ABOVE: Painting on silk, Japan, early nineteenth century
OPPOSITE PAGE, TOP: *Le Viellard et les deux Suzanne,* H.Gerbault
OPPOSITE PAGE, BOTTOM: *The Abbé ,* from Under the Hill, Aubrey Beardsley

Few erotic accoutrements have been quite so successful as the classic combination of stockings and high-heeled shoes. The style of shoe shortens and flatters the foot while lengthening the leg and giving additional height. (It also, incidentally, turns a woman's hips and bottom into an erotic mobile when she walks.) Stockings, whether silk or nylon, give the leg moulding, colour and a clean line. Seamed stockings need more adjustment but the enhanced effect is worth the effort. All of this applies also to tights which are comfortable an practical, but then so are boiler suits. Tights are to stockings as ducks to swans. Legs, after all, are of interest not only in themselves but for where they lead. Stocking-tops, suspenders, thighs and knickers are the Promised Land; tights offer an arid wilderness. In common with men's socks in an erotic context: the sooner they are off, the better.

In the face of universal male disapproval, manufacturers have produced a genuinely erotic idea – crotchless tights. These offer no resistance to a lover's hand; a woman's charms appear as in a vignette, and it is rather like making love through a port-hole: interesting, but hardly a competitor to stockings.

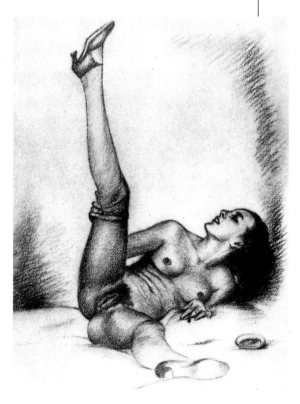

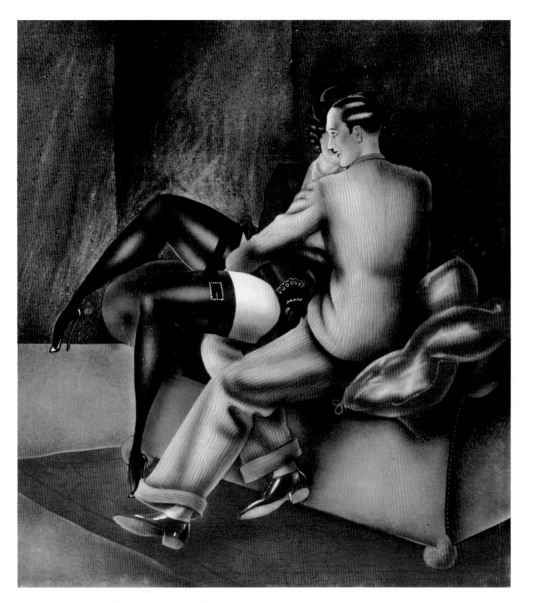

ABOVE: *Fantasy* by 'Carlo', Paris, circa 1930
OPPOSITE PAGE, TOP: Watercolour, Hellmuth Stockmann, circa 1920
OPPOSITE PAGE, BOTTOM: Drawing by an unknown artist, Paris, 1925

Full nakedness! All joys are due to thee;

As souls unbodied, bodies unclothed must be

To taste whole joys...Then, since that I may know,

As liberally as a midwife show

Thyself; cast all, yea, this white linen hence;

There is no penance due to innocence:

To teach thee, I am naked first; why then

What needst thou have more covering than a man?

from *Going to Bed*, John Donne

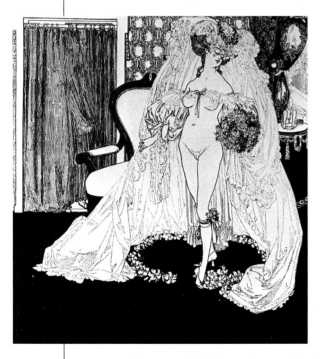

Despite John Donne's entreaties, partial nudity can be highly erotic. In urgent, impassioned lovemaking where we begin fully clothed we are unlikely to remove everything. That is why lingerie is so popular: frou-frou confections to be enjoyed either as they are being removed, or to be lifted or pulled to one side so that they become part of the visual excitement.

Diaphanous clothes can give a grace to the body while allowing tantalising glimpses of its treasures. The more daring society ladies in Regency England rouged their nipples, darkened their pubic hair, and had their maids apply a fine spray of water to heighten the erotic effect.

There is no real male equivalent to this that is not laughable. As a general principle men would do well to follow John Donne's example and remove all their clothes as soon

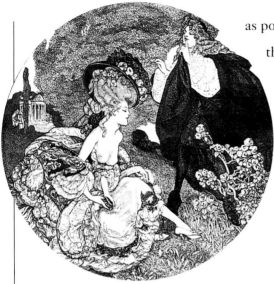

as possible. It is neither good manners nor good sex for the man to be dressed when the woman is not, especially as so many women find it offensive. The minimalist undone fly is acceptable for

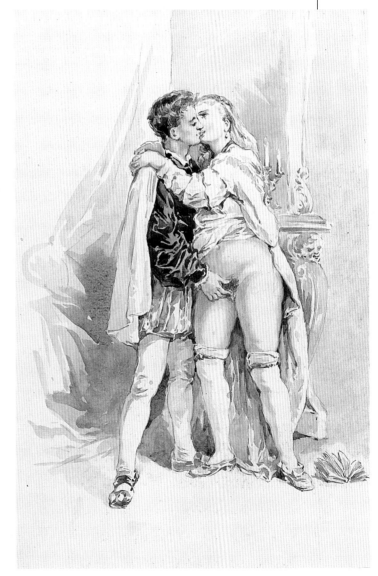

ferocious quickies when neither partner can wait and you risk discovery by ticket collectors or members of the Ramblers' Association. To make a habit of it, as Mussolini did, is boorish.

OPPOSITE PAGE, AND ABOVE: Drawings by Franz von Bayros (1866-1924)
RIGHT: Watercolour attributed to Paul Gavarni (1804-1866)

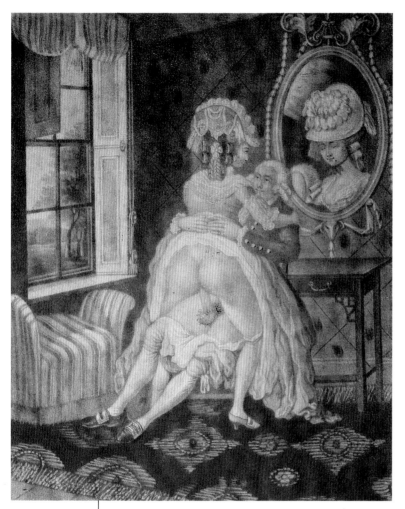

The old-fashioned mirror does not only offer a flawless imitation of life – far better than anything modern technology has yet devised – it is altogether more discreet. This is just as well since mirrors have many erotic applications. Solitary users should remember the fate of Narcissus who fell in love with his own reflection, but no lovers' bedroom can be considered fully furnished without a large mirror. The following humorous episode comes from *The Voluptuous Confessions of a French Lady of Fashion*, a serial published in the Victorian erotic magazine *The Boudoir*. The mirror is not the only witness of the scene...

'With these words she divested herself of her gown, pulled up her shift behind, and placing a big cushion in front of the mirror of the wardrobe, she knelt upon it, her head and arms much lower than her buttocks, which, thrown out and developed by this ravishing position, presented the path of pleasure well in view and largely open. Alfred, far from idle, had made his preparations. He had taken off his jacket and placed the lamp on the floor, so as to light up perfectly the delicious picture that the looking glass reflected in every detail. Then he placed himself behind her, and began to get into her. 'Oh, you can see too much of me!' said my aunt.

'How can I see too much of such beauties? Look in the glass!'

'Oh, no, it's too bad!... Ah!...It's going into me! Stop a little... What a fine fellow you are.'

'My adored one, how lovely you are!' While he spoke he continued his movements. Bertha, in silent enjoyment, said naught, but devoured with eager eye the scene in the glass.'

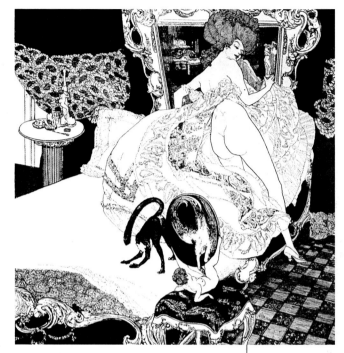

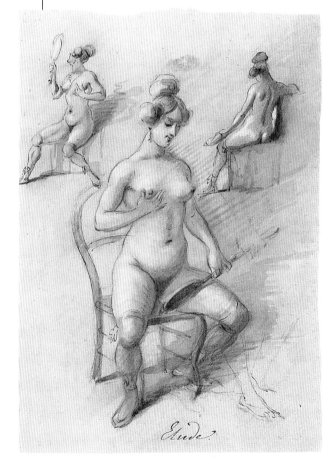

OPPOSITE PAGE: *Rousseau and Madam de Warrens,* from The Confessions, copper engraving, English, eighteenth century
TOP: A book illustration by Franz von Bayros
LEFT: Brush and pen in sepia, French, circa 1780

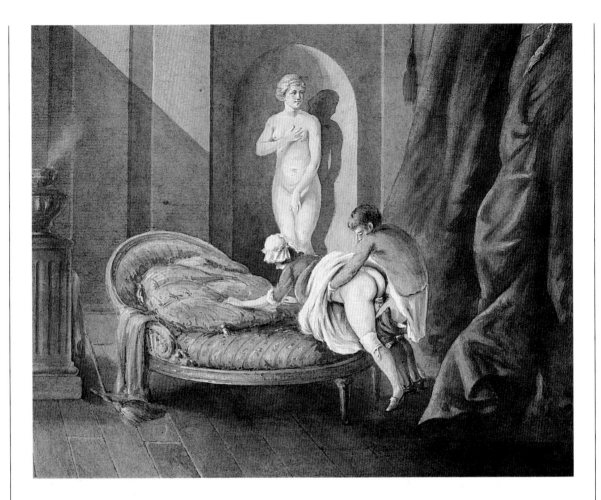

ABOVE: *The Interrupted Work*, Jean Frédéric Schall, 1752-1825
OPPOSITE PAGE, TOP: *Intermezzo*, Léon Adolphe Willette, 1857-1926
OPPOSITE PAGE, BOTTOM: Coloured engraving, anonymous French artist, nineteenth century

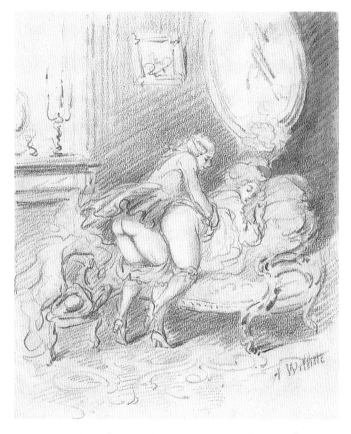

Croupade (rear-entry) and cuissade (straddled) lovemaking postures although the most exciting visually for the man, are less satisfactory in that respect for the woman. Mirrors change this completely, transforming all the rear-entry positions – standing, bending, kneeling, lying flat – into a piece of erotic theatre both can enjoy. Sheikh Nefzawi, author of the great sixteenth-century Arab sex manual *The Perfumed Garden*, suggests a humorous variant which is visually exciting without the use of mirrors: 'Know, oh Vizier, the posture called The Mutual View of the Buttocks. The man lies on his back, and the woman, turning her back to him, sits on his member. He now clasps her body with his legs and she leans over until her hands touch the floor. Thus supported she has a view of his buttocks, and he of hers, and she is able to move conveniently.'

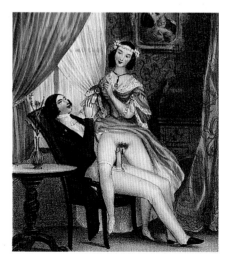

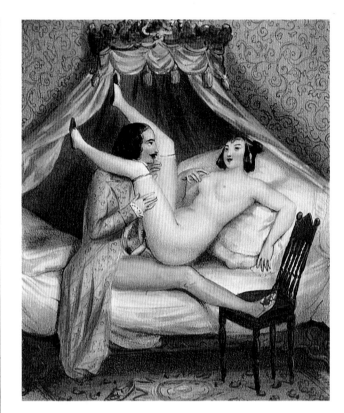

The other series of lovemaking positions which are visually exciting are variants on the X position, and where the woman rides the man – some of the medieval Hindu manuals call this Beauty in Charge. The Kama Sutra of Vatsyanana (1st or 2nd century AD) is more prosaic:

'Women acting the part of a man. There are two ways of doing this, the first is when during congress she turns round, and gets on top of her lover, in such a manner as to continue the congress without obstructing the pleasure of it; and the other is when she acts the man's part from the beginning. At such a time, with flowers in her hair hanging loose, and her smiles broken by hard breathings, she should press upon her lover's bosom with her own breasts, and lowering her head frequently, should do in return the same actions which he used to do before '

ABOVE: Coloured engraving, anonymous French artist, nineteenth century
OPPOSITE PAGE: *The Red Armchair,* Louis Jaugey, circa 1870

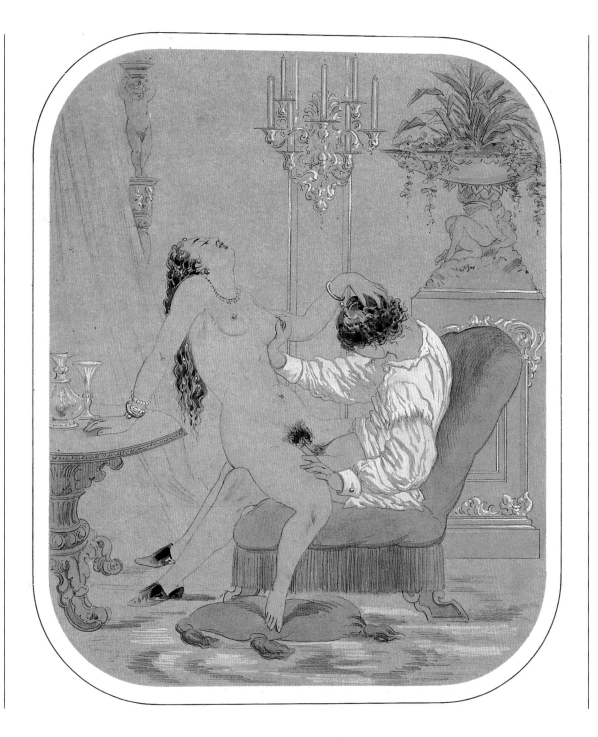

Erotic art is a celebration of our sexuality and is, in that sense, a 'mirror held up to life'. To be offended and shocked by skilful representations of sex and nudity is to deny an important part of our humanity and to miss out on a lot of fun. The arabesques lovers see their bodies making in bedroom mirrors are exciting: they increase the pleasure they have in one another. To see others making love is exciting too, and erotic art gives us that possibility. Some of the very first images in art, from as early a s 30,000 BC, are sexual. Providing that the sexual energy generated is channelled back into life and does not become a voyeuristic end in itself, erotic art is as useful as it is pleasurable. Art, like Alice's looking glass, opens into another world. Erotic art is as infinite and varied as human imagination, a vehicle for every kind of fantasy. That can be useful and enjoyable too, providing it gives something back to life and is not pernicious or cruel. Artists whose erotic vision is 'through a glass darkly' are to be avoided.

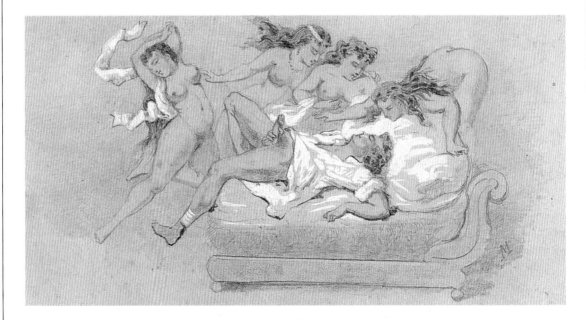

OPPOSITE PAGE: *L'Art et La Vie,* Walter Crane, 1845-1915
ABOVE: *The Dream,* Henry Monnier, 1799-1875

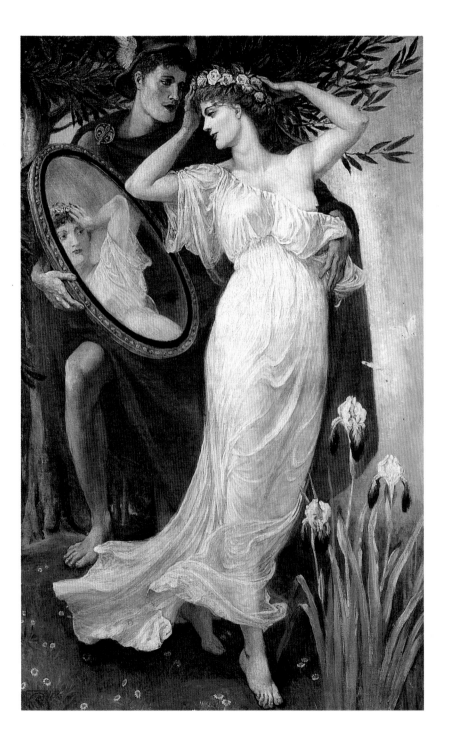

Visual erotica can be instructive as well as beautiful. Indian miniaturists illustrated sexual postures from the Hindu love manuals and Japanese shunga prints were an important feature of the eighteenth-century 'pillow books' of erotic instruction. The lady in the woodblock print opposite has been moved to artistic as well as to sexual expression, and is practising calligraphy on her lover's penis! In the West, Pietro Aretino (1492-1557) wrote sonnets to accompany engravings made from the famous 'postures' which the artist Giulio Romano (1550-1618) had drawn on a wall in the Vatican. These sixteen positions, copied and re-copied by numerous artists, were part of the sexual education of the privileged in the seventeenth and eighteenth centuries. We know from his *Mémoires* that Casanova used them to excite and instruct new conquests.

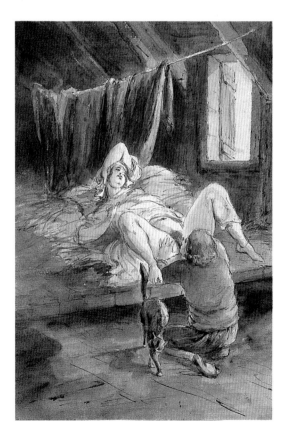 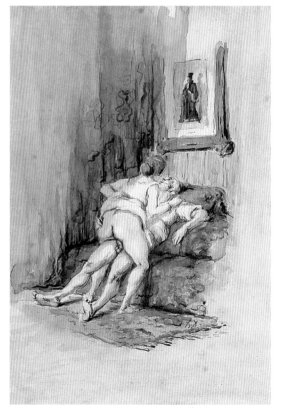

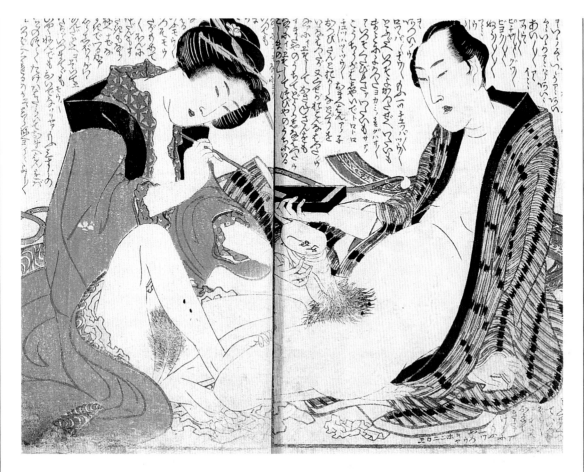

ABOVE: Shunga print, Japan, late-eighteenth century
OPPOSITE PAGE, FAR LEFT: Sepia drawing, French, artist unknown
OPPOSITE PAGE, LEFT: *Home Pleasures*, Honoré Daumier, 1808-1879

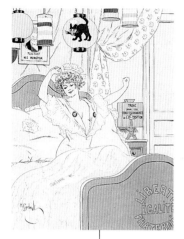

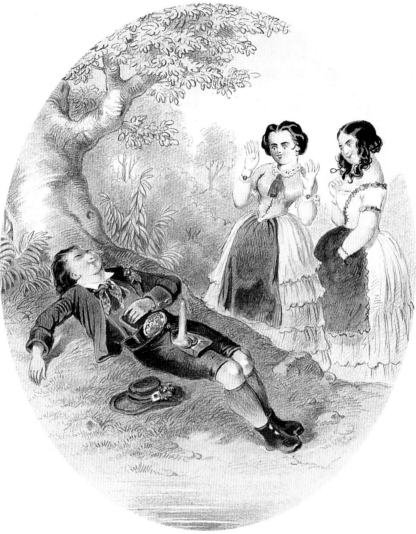

OPPOSITE PAGE: French postcards, circa 1900
French lithograph, circa 1880
ABOVE: Coloured print, anonymous German artist, nineteenth century
TOP: *L'Exposition est close*, H.Gerbault, Paris

Humorous erotica – often vulgar in tone – became increasingly popular during the nineteenth century. Publishers were able to exploit the new printing technology by selling rude postcards and erotic prints to the railway tourists who flooded into Europe's capitals to visit the great exhibitions. Variable in the quality of art, printing – and humour – the mass market erotica of the Age of Travel is nevertheless a useful reminder of the lighter side of sexuality.

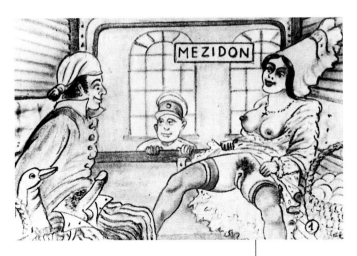

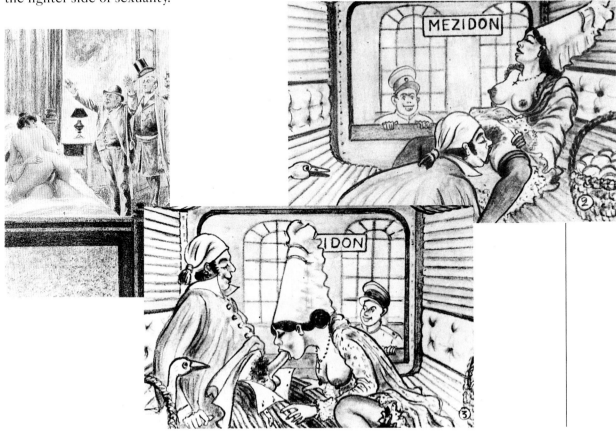

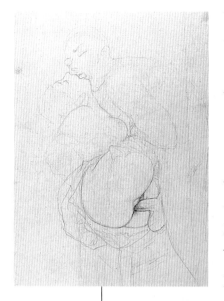

Travel is one of life's great pleasures. To be in love anywhere is
wonderful. To be in Paris, or Venice, or under the blue skies of the
Mediterranean and in love, is as near to heaven as the living can get.
The elusive 'spirit of place' is of course a combination of many different
sensory impressions and associations, but light is paramount. It is not
necessary to be an artist to enjoy the intense sensual pleasure light can
give, it is there for all to see. In autumn, Venice's architectural glories are
lit from above and more subtly from below, where the milky opalescent
light is reflected back from the waters of the canals and lagoon. New
York on a clear winter's morning is like steel being cut with acetylene.
London – largely because of the airport, but what matter – has great

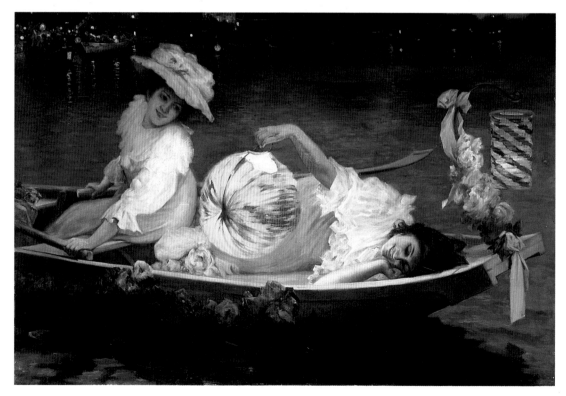

aching sunsets towards the end of summer.

Travel is a pleasure lovers can enjoy together if they are fortunate. But everything is a gift of the light, including the ability to see each other. The human face changes in candlelight; the naked body is never more beautiful than in the warmth of fire light.

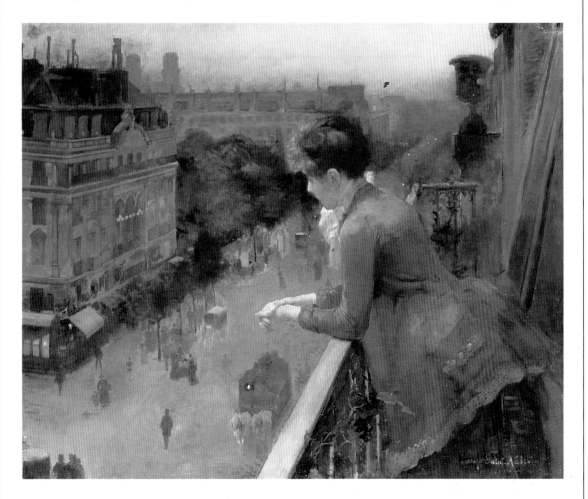

ABOVE: *A Young Lady Looking Towards the Chatelet, Paris,* Charles Leroy-Saint Aubert, born 1856
OPPOSITE PAGE, BOTTOM: *Dreaming,* Ulpiano Checa y Sanz, 1860-1916
OPPOSITE PAGE, TOP: Pencil drawing by an unknown Italian artist

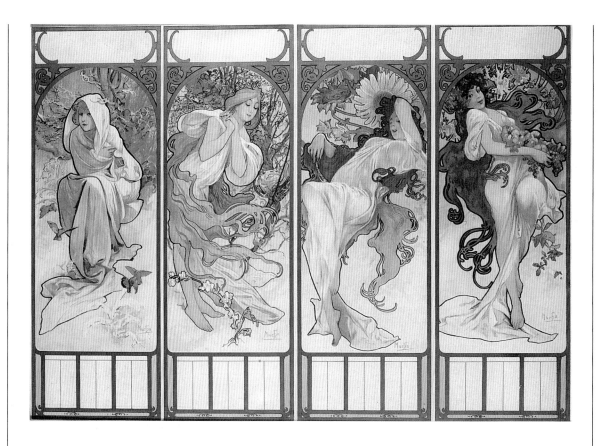

ABOVE: *Calendar of the Four Seasons,* Alfons Mucha, 1860-1939
OPPOSITE PAGE: *In the Cornfield,* Michel Martin Drolling, 1786-1851

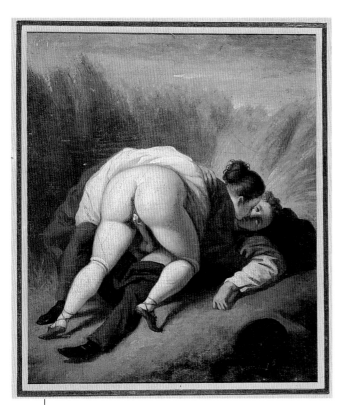

If we are fortunate enough to live in a climate where there are four distinct seasons, we can enjoy the changing intensity of sunlight and all that comes with that: the different temperatures and vegetation, and of course the different moods.

The seasons are also the most powerful metaphor we have for the changes which take place in ourselves as the years pass, changes we must also learn to enjoy. We cannot live in perpetual glorious spring and just as well; April is indeed 'the cruelest month,' the sensations we experience often painful in their intensity. A long summer in which to enjoy all the adult pleasures is the greatest blessing a man and a woman can hope for. Then, after days of blazing sunshine, a mellow autumn has its proper place:

> No Spring nor summer beauty hath such grace,
> As I have seen in one Autumnal face.
>
> John Donne

Winter too comes in its right time. Not a season for regrets – unless of course we wasted life, and did not enjoy summer to the full.

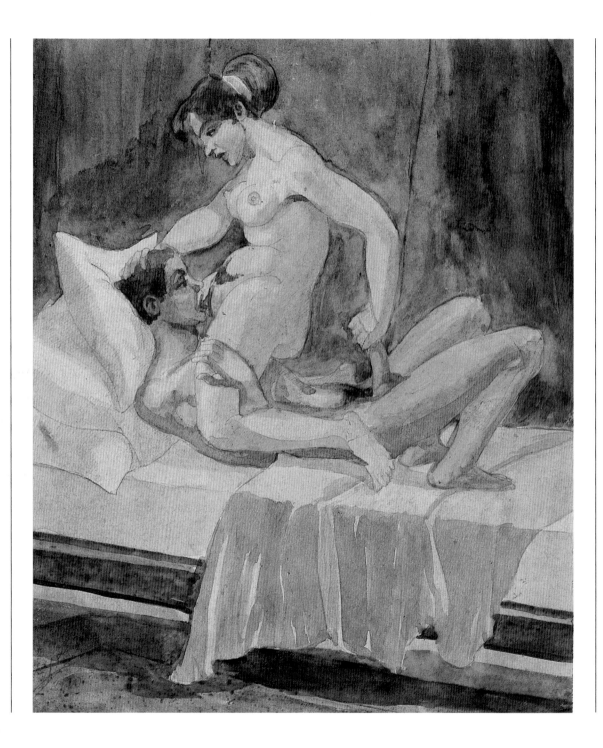

TASTE

Her breath is like honey spiced with cloves,
Her mouth delicious as a ripened mango.
To press kisses on her skin is to taste the lotus,
The deep cave of her navel hides a store of spices
What pleasure lies beyond, the tongue knows,
But cannot speak of it.

Srngarakarika, Kumaradatta (12th century AD)

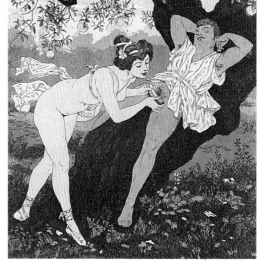

With lips and tongue, and the moist suction of our mouths, we can both give and receive enormous pleasure. The concentration of sensitive nerve endings which respond to touch and temperature, and taste buds which can detect salt, sour, sweet and bitter essences, make the mouth a uniquely gifted lover: a Casanova and a Cleopatra; a Falstaff and an eroticized Mrs Beeton.

OPPOSITE PAGE: A Watercolour by the Hungarian artist 'Fay D', Paris circa 1920
ABOVE: Lithograph intended as a book illustration, artist unknown

A kiss upon the lips can be the gentle token of affection or the expression of a burning passion. At its most extreme, in maraichinage or 'French kissing', tongue and mouth become surrogate sexual organs in an orgy of reciprocal thrusts. Vatsyayana has much to say on the subject of kissing in *Kama Sutra*:

'When a man kisses the upper lip of a woman, while she in return kisses his lower lip, it is called the 'kiss of the upper'.

When one of them takes both the lips of the other between his or her own, it is called a 'clasping kiss'. A woman, however, only takes this kind of kiss from a man with no moustache. And on the occasion of this kiss, if one of them touches the teeth, the tongue, and the palate of the other, with his or her tongue, it is called the 'fighting of the tongue.'

A thousand years after Vatsyayana finished compiling *Kama Sutra*, the great Arab erotologist Sheikh Nefzawi gives his views on kissing in *The Perfumed Garden*:

'Believe me, kisses, nibblings, sucking of lips, close-clasping of breasts, and the drinking of passion-loaded spittle, are the things which ensure a durable affection.'

OPPOSITE PAGE: Mythological scene, after Paolo Farinato, 1524-1606
BELOW: *By the Roadside*, Mihaly Zichy, 1827-1906

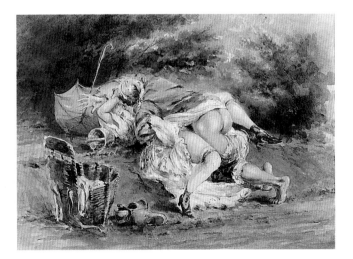

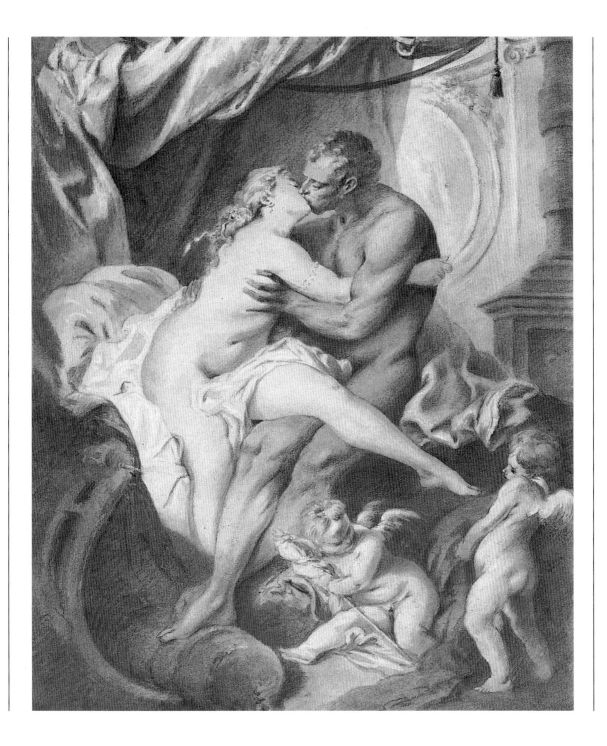

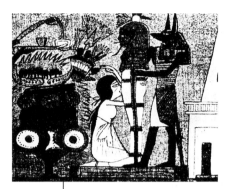

Fellatio – exciting the penis by licking and sucking – is as old as mankind. In all periods and all cultures men have enjoyed fellatio, and the women generous enough to indulge them have wished that their jaws did not ache quite so much. Cleopatra's skill in fellatio was famed throughout the Roman world. In *Kama Sutra* it is called the 'auparishtaka' or Mouth Congress; this description is from the medieval Hindu text *Ratiratnapradipika*:

'Her mouth quickens now upon the shaft; when you
                                    stir to her lips
and tongue-tip, she swallows it as deeply as
                                    she can and kisses
when you cry out: this is Sangara, Swallowed Up.'

In *My Life and Loves*, Lorna Mayhew gives the young Frank Harris some useful insights as well as a good time:

'She began here to breathe more quickly. 'I've been thinking how to give you more pleasure; let me try. Your seed, darling, is dear to me: I don't want it in my sex; I want to feel you thrill and so I want your sex in my mouth, I want to drink your essence and I will '– and suiting the action to the word, she slipped down in the bed and took my sex in her mouth and began rubbing it up and down till my seed spirted in long jets, filling her mouth while she swallowed it greedily. 'Now do I love, Sir!' she exclaimed... 'Wait till some girl does that to you and you'll know she loves you to distraction... '

ABOVE: Tomb Painting, Upper Egypt, date unknown
OPPOSITE PAGE: Coloured lithograph, Circle of Achille Devéria, 1800-1875

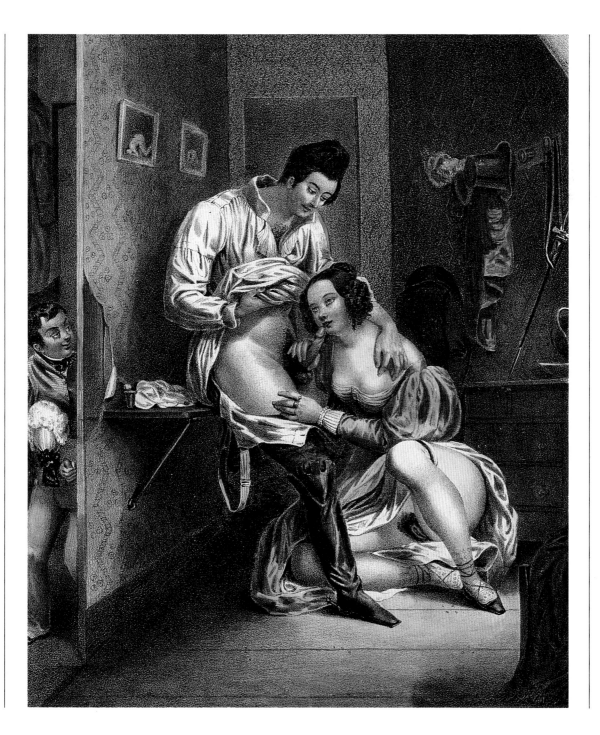

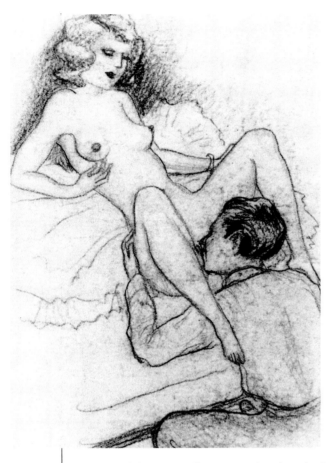

Cunnilingus – where the vulva is stimulated by the tongue and lips – is as indispensable in lovemaking as fellatio, perhaps more indispensable. Fellatio requires considerable skill and flair: an erotic drama with several players including a temperamental male lead. Cunnilingus (in reality a play for two actors: tongue and clitoris) should be regarded as an essential and regular feature of the repertoire. With the difference in male and female sexual response, cunnilingus is a woman's insurance: a delightful way of guaranteeing an orgasm.

This extract is taken from *Story of O* by Pauline Réage; only two protagonists are involved:

'For nigh on to an hour Jacqueline moaned under O's caresses, and finally, her nipples erected, her arms flung over her head, clutching the wooden bars at the head of her bed, she began to scream when O dividing the lips fringed with pale hair, set quietly and slowly to biting the tiny inflamed morsel of flesh protruding from the cowl formed by the juncture of those sweet and delicate little labia. O felt it heat and rise under her tongue, and, nipping mercilessly, fetched cry after cry from Jacqueline until she broke like a pane of glass, and relaxed, soaked from joy.'

ABOVE: Pencil drawing by 'AI', Vienna, 1935
OPPOSITE PAGE, TOP: *The Red Hat,* 'Barlog', Berlin circa 1930
OPPOSITE PAGE, BOTTOM: Anonymous watercolour, Italy, circa 1930

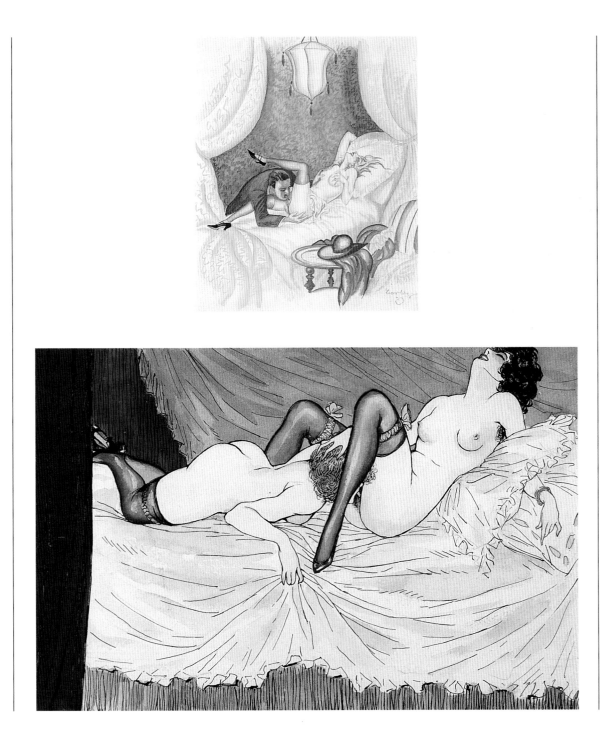

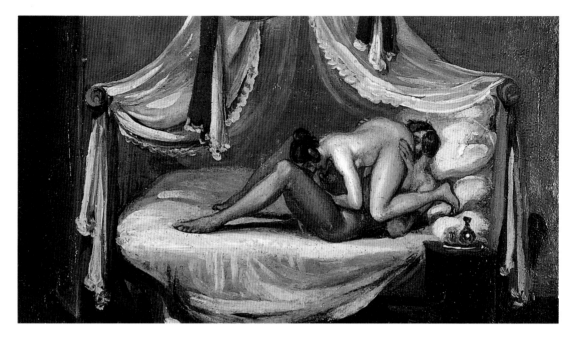

ABOVE: Anonymous oil painting, French, eighteenth century
BELOW: Watercolour by an unknown Italian artist, circa 1930

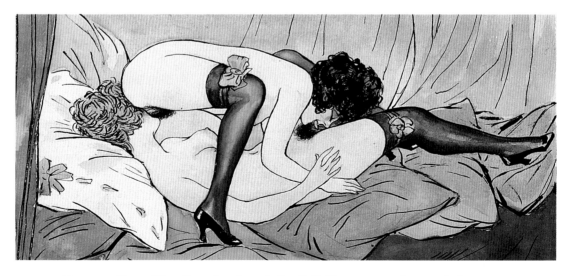

OPPOSITE PAGE, TOP: Drawing, Joseph Ortoloff, Germany, early twentieth century
OPPOSITE PAGE, BOTTOM: *'69'*, Victorian erotic postcard

Orality involves our lips and tongues in an erotic exploration of our lover: the different shapes and textures of helmet and shaft, of clitoris and labia. In doing this we can also enjoy the tastes of each other (and the scents, which we will be dealing with later). The sexual fluids of both men and women are highly individual and change their taste dramatically according to mood and other factors. As a connoisseur and regular taster of your lover you will, however, detect a consistent style to the products of his or her private domain.

Soixante-neuf – the inverted posture with either partner on top or both comfortably side by side – is the ideal position for comparative tastings. This description of '69' is taken from *Passion's Apprentice:*

'… she swung her leg across his chest and, bending, took him in her mouth. The sensation of her sucking at him, and her hair dancing on his thighs as she rocked to and fro, was almost unbearable in its intensity.

He raised his head. Her sex was like a delicate sea shell, the palest pink fading into

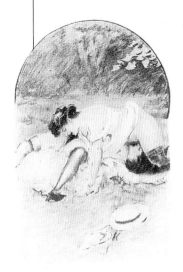

white. It opened each time she rocked forward, while above her buttocks parted and disclosed a tiny pink rose.

He groaned as she took him deeper in her mouth, moving more urgently. The pleasure began like a thrill deep inside him, rising nearer and nearer to the surface … At last it was released. That was the crisis of his pleasure, that and her soft mouth sucking the pumping shaft and drinking him.

She kissed him slowly on the lips. Her breath was like new mown grass. 'I love the taste of you'.

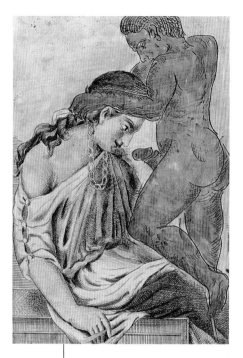

Gastronomy competes with sex in the number of senses it stimulates. In addition to pleasing the eye and nose, food should stimulate the mouth with interesting shapes and textures. The Japanese passion for raw fish is as much to do with the enormous variety of texture provided by seafood as with its taste. In a well-planned menu a sequence of tastes in which each new arrival contrasts pleasantly with the last is the ideal. Temperatures can be contrasted in the same way. A meal then becomes similar to a musical composition, with a series of structured crescendos. Unfortunately there is a tendency for 'refined' cuisine to concentrate on the taste and appearance of food and to ignore texture. This expensive and over-prepared baby food should be avoided.

The intimate links between sex and eating – based upon complicated associations involving all the senses – turn the dining table into a bed, and the bed into a dining table. Seafood is sexy. Shellfish in particular seem to have been designed by an erotomaniac with an interest in surrealism. Mussels expose themselves to us in steamy sauna tureens, and day-trippers put vinegar on cockle clitorises by the seaside. While nibbling a scallop nipple, or slipping a lobster claw penis between our lips, we should remember that aeons ago we came from the sea. That is why our most intimate secretions are salty, smelling and tasting of the ocean, and why fruits de mer is such a sensual – and sexual – treat.

ABOVE: Anonymous coloured engraving
OPPOSITE PAGE, BOTTOM: *The Feast of Neptune*, Hendrick Van Balen, seventeenth century
OPPOSITE PAGE, TOP: *Still life with prawns*, Edward Ladell, 1821-1886

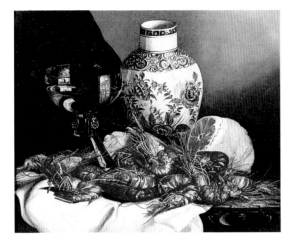

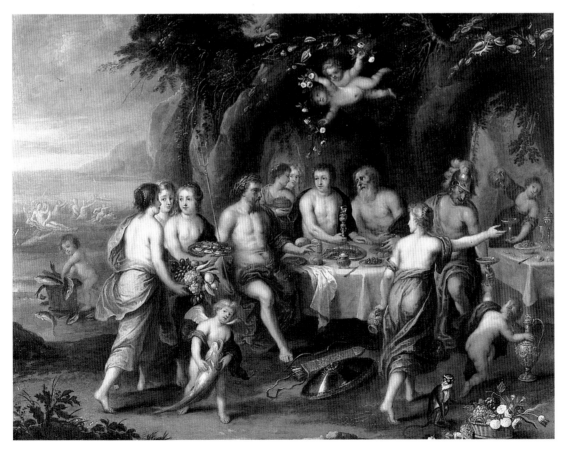

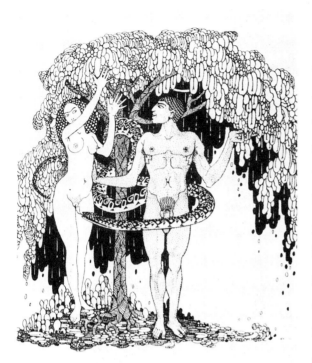

Foods which are popularly regarded as 'aphrodisiacs' often rely upon the conscious and unconscious associations we make between sex and food. Asparagus is phallic in shape and has a pungent, evocative aroma. The eating of asparagus – a sort of symbolic fellatio – may either stir unconscious erotic thoughts, or conscious sexual jokes. In either case bed is one step nearer. Nature is a lascivious old pander who has provided our larder with innumerable phallic fruits and vegetables from the mushroom to the cucumber. It was never quite clear whether the popular marketing slogan 'unzip a banana' was a conscious or unconscious double entendre.

Aphrodisiacs which mimic female sexual organs in the endlessly fecund human imagination are also numerous. Pomegranates were burst open at Chinese weddings and eaten at the Dionysiac orgies in ancient Greece. Figs and watermelons have the same erotic associations.

In Classical times sex was never far from the table. Worshippers of Aphrodite in Syracuse baked vulva-shaped bread, while the ever-erect Priapus was celebrated with the phallic loaves which French boulangers still make today.

Oysters, which have been regarded as aphrodisiacs since Roman times, are more difficult to decode. They have the slightly salty sea taste which is exciting and evocative for both men and woman. But it is the sheer sensuality of eating an oyster that is the secret of its erotic reputation. Casanova, Chevalier de Seingalt (1725-1798) managed to seduce two young nuns together by plying them with oysters and champagne.

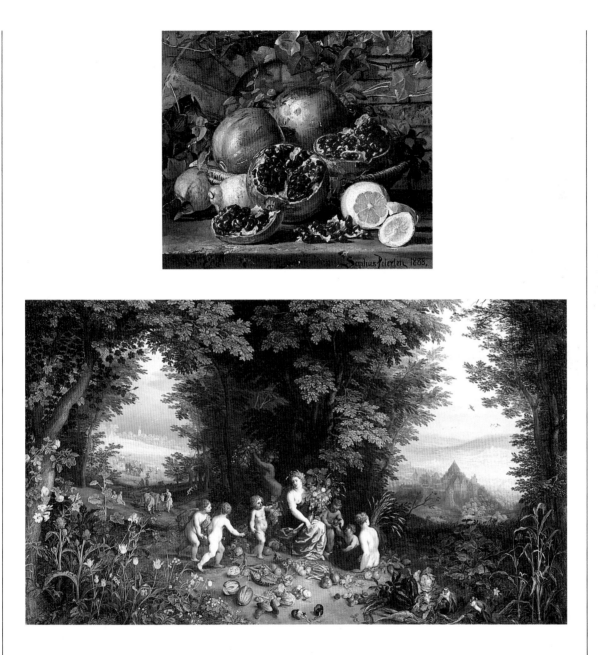

TOP: Still Life, Magnus Otto Sophus Petersen, 1837-1904
BOTTOM: *Earth,* Jan Breughel, 1568-1625
OPPOSITE PAGE: *Adam & Eve*, drawing by an unknown artist, twentieth century

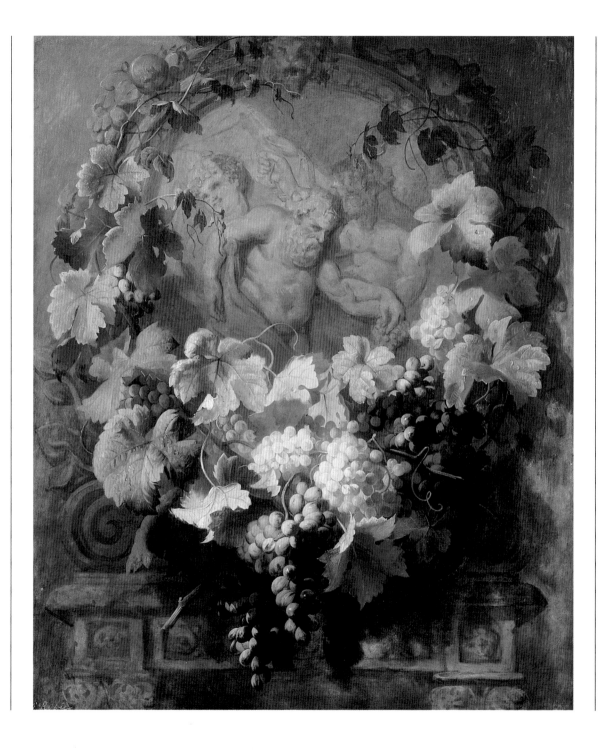

Sine Baccho et Cerere frigescit Venus – 'without Bacchus (the vine) and Ceres (the harvest) Venus (love) is cold.'

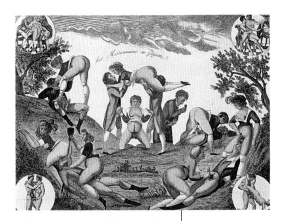

Wine is a sensual pleasure, one as old as civilization. Just as Bacchus often kept company with Pan and his libidinous satyrs, so wine and love make a perfect match. Champagne is often the choice of lovers, and with good reason. It is a lively, exciting wine: its bubbles thrill lips, mouth and tongue, and then carry its alcohol quickly into the bloodstream. It is always drunk chilled, and the kisses of champagne-cold lips on warm flesh are erotic 'coups de rapier'. Soft, round red wines – like the apotheosis of Valpolicella, amarone; or Zinfandel, or the spicy shiraz creations of Australian wine makers – are ideal for winter lovemaking in front of the fire. But the most erotic wines are those made from the muscat grape. A journalist visiting a cellar in Moravia, stuck for words, asked the old cellarman how he would describe one particularly sensuous muscat. Without hesitation this grinning Silenus told him to recall the scent of a sexually excited woman: a description as perfect as it was difficult for the earnest translator!

Muscat grapes are made into an extraordinary variety of quite different wines, all retaining the unique perfume. In Alsace, muscat grapes become a delicate, dry aperitif wine; in Beaumes de Venise a scented, sweet dessert wine; in Italy delicious sparkling Moscato d'Asti.

Sensualists and romantics in search of the ultimate erotic wine – erotic in itself and the perfect drink for lovers – should try Hungarian Tokay. This is the legendary wine of kings and emperors, a precious nectar so pure it is reputed to last for centuries.

ABOVE: *The Envoys on a Spree*, French coloured engraving, late-eighteenth century
OPPOSITE PAGE: *A Tribute to Bacchus*, Jean-Baptiste Robie, 1821-1910

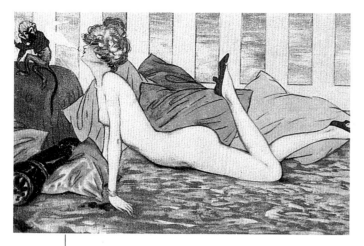

Smoking is an expression of our orality, although the sultan in the illustration seems to have abandoned the joys of his hubbly-bubbly in favour of a different kind of oral gratification. Quite apart from the tastes, smells and chemical stimulation which tobacco provides, it is pleasant to stimulate the lips and tongue physically. That is why people who give up smoking often eat more or take to drinking numerous cups of coffee.

The negative effects of smoking are very real and potentially dangerous, and it is good that we are now aware of them. But smoking is not automatically a 'dirty habit' as the puritans would have us believe. If we are not fastidious we can certainly make it a dirty habit, but then we can do that to many other activities. Handled stylishly, the rituals of smoking are rather elegant; a cigarette, cigar or pipe an interesting addition to face or hands, with its spiralling plume of grey-blue smoke.

Fine tobacco is delicious if you like it. Cigarette tobacco ranges from mild, sweet Virginia leaf, to dark, aromatic Balkan blends. Pipe smokers have an almost infinite variety to choose from, including blends that have been soaked in molasses and other substances. The Havana cigar, with its uniquely mild flavour and heady incense-like aroma, has often been described as a phallic symbol. But as Freud himself remarked 'sometimes a cigar is just a cigar'.

ABOVE: Coloured lithograph, early twentieth century
OPPOSITE PAGE: *The Sultan,* anonymous book illustration circa 1930

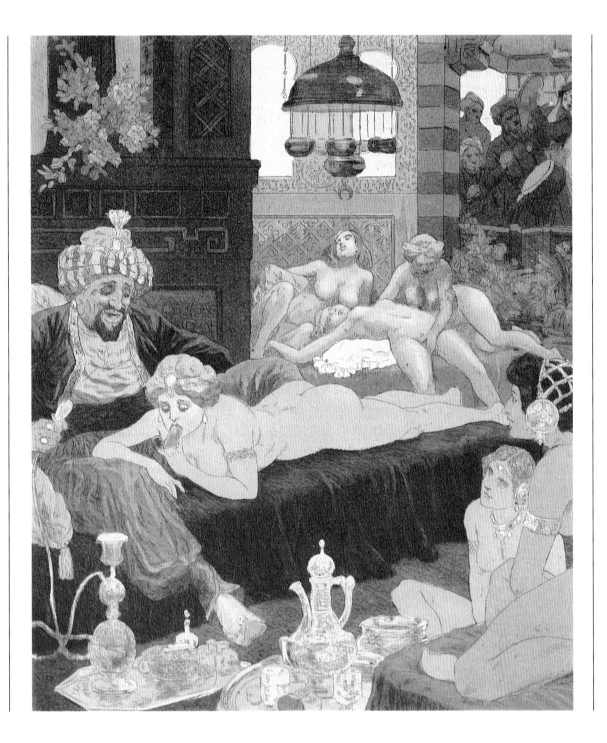

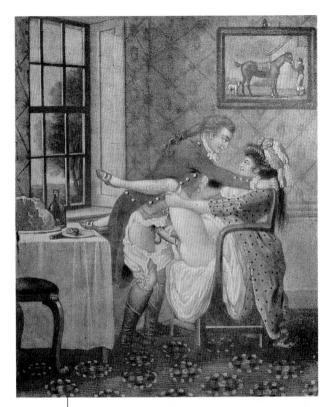

In Jean Cocteau's astonishingly beautiful film of Beauty and the Beast (*La Belle et la Bête*, 1946) we are struck by the impeccable manners of the Beast. The sight of his hairy male animality contained by eighteenth-century clothes and the rules of gentle behaviour is both touching and sexy. So potent is the magic, that when the Beast is finally transformed into Prince Charming we rather resent the new arrival and regret the disappearance of the courteous Beast.

Manners, table manners especially, are largely an inheritance from the Victorians. It is a useful inheritance: dining is one of life's great pleasures because of the rituals associated with what is, at its most basic, an animal requirement. We shall have a lot to say in this book about the balance between animality and civilized behaviour, since this is the essence of sensuality.

Dining with a lover is enjoyable both in itself and because of the erotic pleasures for which it is an overture. The oral pleasure of eating and the symbolism involved also anticipate to some degree the enjoyment to come. This has never been more vividly illustrated than by the dining scene in another film: Tony Richardson's *Tom Jones* (1963). In the eighteenth-century illustration from Fielding's novel shown here, Tom and Mrs Waters seem to have reached the post-prandial stage.

OPPOSITE PAGE, BOTTOM: *Au Restaurant le Doyen*, Ernest Ange Duiz, Paris, circa 1878
ABOVE: *Tom Jones and Mrs Waters*, copper engraving, eighteenth century
OPPOSITE PAGE, TOP: Decorated entrée dish, China, nineteenth century

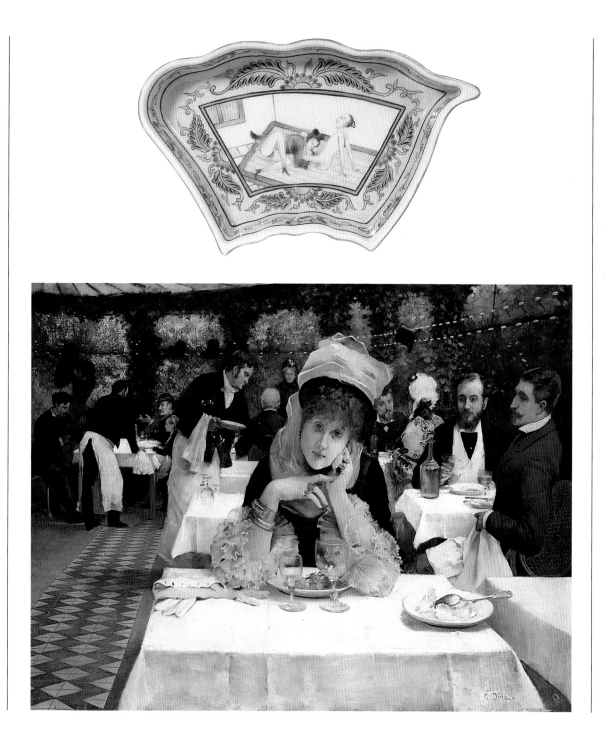

The reciprocity between table and bed is so great that we can learn a good deal of a person's sexual manners from their eating habits. Someone who pays no attention to anyone else's plate or glass is likely to be selfish in bed; nor is slovenliness such as nose blowing at table or eating with the mouth open a good augury. Victorian table manners are concerned with making eating aesthetically pleasing. The moderated form in which this etiquette survives is concerned with enjoyment not repression: table linen is not fussy (or should not be) but highly sensual.

The sensuality of the Victorian age – all the more powerful and pervasive for being contained – found open expression in their gastronomy. Isabella Beeton's *Book of Household Management* (1861) is to cooking what *Kama Sutra* is to sex (if that sounds fanciful, read them). But the most sensual Victorian book on gastronomy is *Kettner's Book of the Table* by E.S.Dallas (1871). It is an amusing and scholarly book, full of anecdotes such as the story of the great chef Vatel who killed himself when the turbot failed to arrive, and jokes such as 'brownings are as admirable in soup as Robert Browning in poesy – but they are apt to be harsh.' To eat veal, according to Dallas, 'is as insipid as kissing one's sister'.

Dallas was the chief book reviewer and obituarist (Palmerston, Thackeray, Prince Albert) for *The Times*; the friend of Dickens, George Eliot, Rossetti and Landseer. His sensuality was his downfall; in the end he was ruined by scandal:

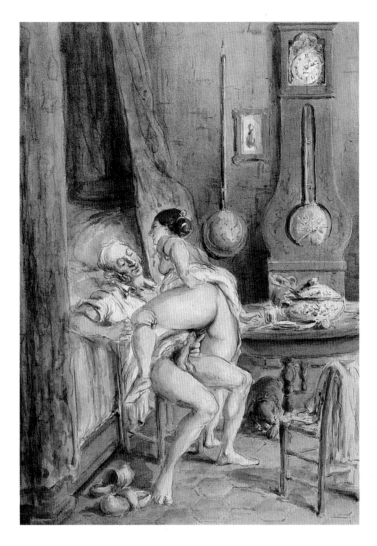

'Poor old Dallas!

All along of his phallus,

Must he come to the gallows?'

OPPOSITE PAGE: Chinese export tableware for the European market, nineteenth century
ABOVE: Pen and Watercolour, circle of Honoré Daumier

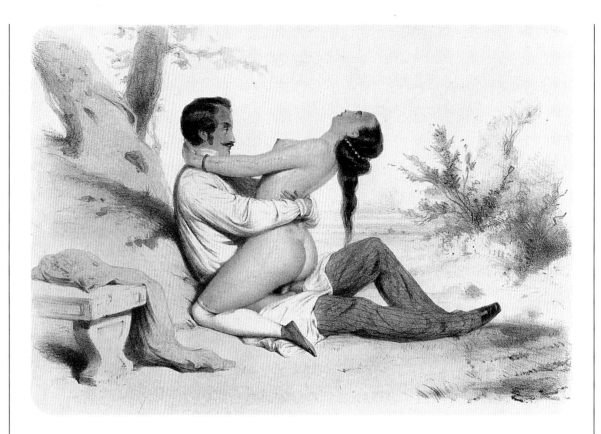

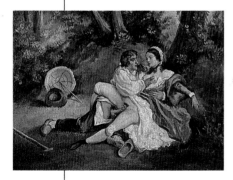

During the nineteenth century the idea of eating outdoors – the picnic – became increasingly popular. And, as we have already seen, eating is often the overture to other pleasures. Romanticism, with its idealization of nature and the countryside, is a potent force, drawing as it does upon the deep well of our collective unconscious. The sensual urge to be outdoors, to eat, sleep and of course make love outdoors, is part of our animal inheritance – a factor which will play an increasingly important part when as we examine the next sense, Smell.

'She was nearly at the wide riding when he came up and flung his naked arm round her soft, naked-wet middle. She gave a shriek and straightened herself, and the heap of her soft, chill flesh came up against his body. He pressed it all up against him, madly, the heap of soft, chilled, female flesh that became quickly warm as flame, in contact. The rain streamed on them till they smoked. He gathered her lovely, heavy posteriors one in each hand and pressed them in towards him in a frenzy, quivering motionless in the rain. Then suddenly he tipped her up and fell with her on the path, in the roaring silence of the rain, and short and sharp, he took her, short and sharp and finished, like an animal.'

Lady Chatterley's Lover, D.H.Lawrence (1885-1930)

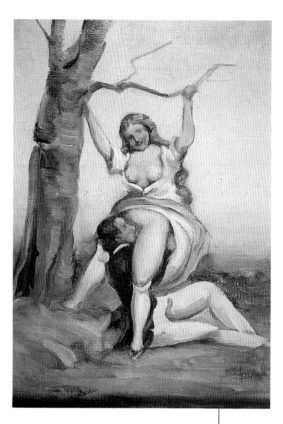

ABOVE: *The Interrupted Walk in the Woods,* Achille Devéria, 1800-1857
OPPOSITE PAGE, TOP: *Chemin faisant,* anonymous coloured engraving, nineteenth century
OPPOSITE PAGE, BOTTOM: Oil painting by an unknown artist, nineteenth century

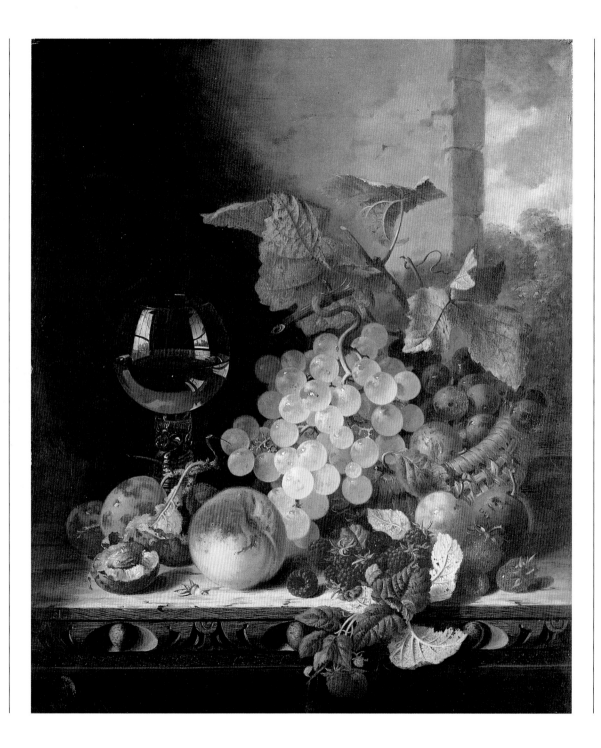

SMELL

The position of the human nose was not an arbitrary design decision (although in some cases it may appear so) but the result of aeons of evolution. Our organ of smell is placed above the organ concerned with taste, the mouth, because of the intimate link between the two: no other two senses have such a close relationship. In activities where taste and smell are both involved – for example wine, food or sex – it may be hard to decide which sense gives us the greater pleasure, although smell is infinitely more powerful and discriminating than taste. Our sense of smell has unique access to the brain: we can detect a scent even before we can feel pain. The brain itself developed from the olfactory bulb, and the ancient channel to it has carried information about the smells in the world around us since that world was the primordial ocean.

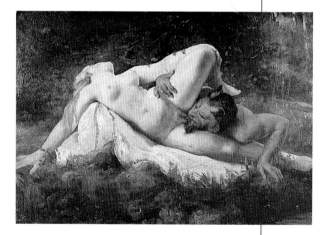

OPPOSITE PAGE: *Still Life,* Edward Ladell, 1821-1886
ABOVE: *Nymph & Satyr,* Artur Fischer, 1872-1948

One of Sigmund Freud's disciples, Sandor Ferenczi, developed a theory that the fishy odours associated with the genitals were the key to understanding the sexual urge, which he believed was driven by a desire to return to the Cambrian seas from which all life came. *Thalassa: a theory of genitality,* may be difficult reading for non-Freudians, but it does shed light on what is – to use one of Freud's own terms – a taboo subject. Our genitals do have a maritime air about them: the penis of a naked man walking even has the rolling gait of a sailor. Fishy odours are common and natural even if we are healthy

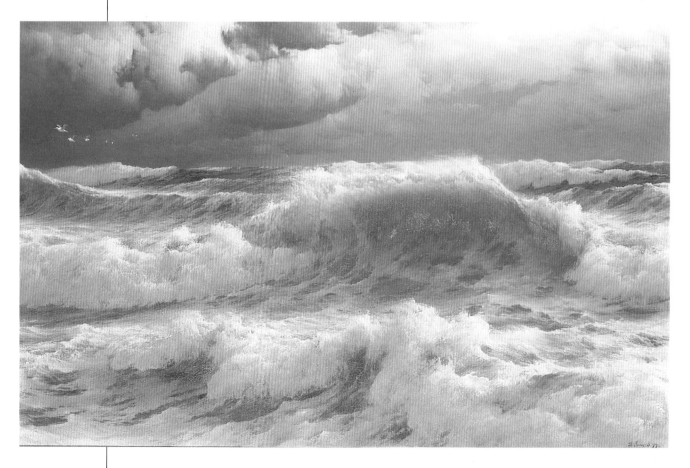

OPPOSITE PAGE: *Goldfische,* Gustav Klimt, 1901/2
ABOVE: *Seascape,* David James, 1897

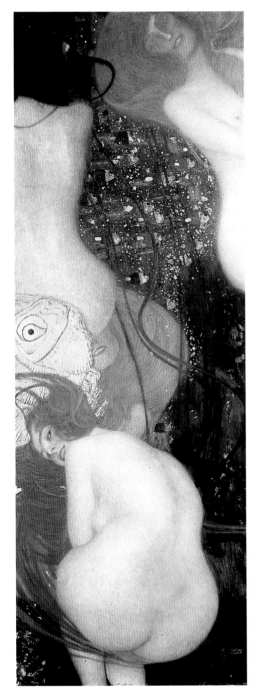

and bathe regularly. Sexual fluids are saline, as are the secretions we produce to keep the membranes of our nose moist in order that we can retain the ability to smell.

The human body is composed mainly of water and it needs salt in order to survive. All this is uncontentious biological fact: our ancestors did at some point aeons ago, and for reasons best known to themselves, crawl out of the ocean and our bodies reflect that. Whether we want to return to the sea – except for holidays – is more controversial. But there is little point in shedding (saline) tears at our fishy inheritance.

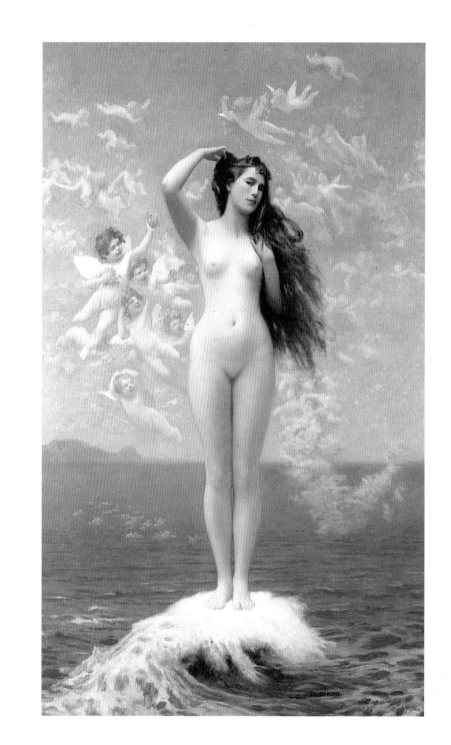

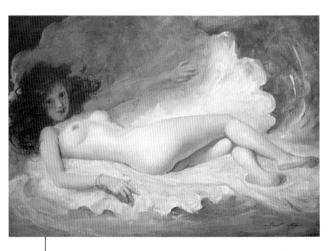

It is no coincidence that the goddess of Love herself, Aphrodite, came from the sea. Her name means 'surf born'. The seductive sea nymphs – of whom there are more than three thousand in Classical mythology – make their own case for the marine aspects of female sexual attraction. Most unambiguous of all are the delightful mermaids, who have little choice but to come to terms with biology.

There is a point in calling to the witness stand half the characters in Classical mythology in order to discuss a woman's natural scent. There are those who would have us ashamed of our bodies instead of celebrating the fact that we have natural aromas which are vital in sexual attraction and a source of sensual pleasure. Emile Zola (1840-1902) well understood the importance of our sense of smell in sexual relations, it is a theme he returns to again and again in his novels. In *Nana*, the heroine decides to use her 'strong female odour' destructively, as 'a force of Nature'. Zola describes the plot of this sensual, atmospheric book as 'the cunt in all its power; the cunt as an altar with all men offering up their sacrifices to it. The book is the poem of the cunt…'

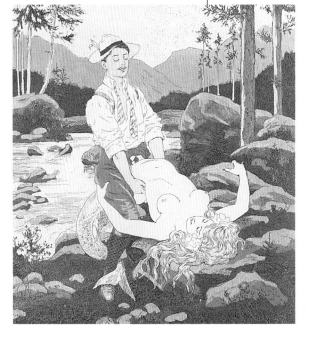

OPPOSITE PAGE: *Venus Rising from the Waves,* J.L. Gerome, nineteenth century
TOP: *Nymph,* Szantho Maria, Hungary, nineteenth century
BOTTOM: *The Mermaid,* book illustration, anonymous.

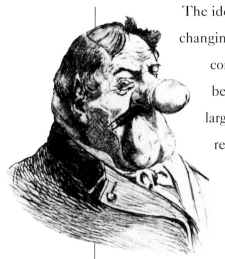

The identification of the nose with the penis is very old. Small boys have been changing drawings of one to the other certainly since Roman times when it was commonplace in graffiti. At least as ancient is the supposed correlation between the size of nose and penis, and Ovid (who presumably had a large nose) pronounced 'Noscitur e naso quanta sit hasta viro.' With the renaissance of such Classical wisdom there must have been many disappointments in fourteenth-century Italy.

In sixteenth-century England the dramatist Philip Massinger (1583-1640) refers to a supposed connection between a woman's nose and her sexual appetite:

'Her nose, which by its length assures me
Of storms at midnight if I fail to pay her
The tributes she expects.'

Nose-sex correlations may be unreliable for predicting either penile size or female appetite, but there are physiological links between noses and sexuality. Perhaps because our sense of smell becomes more efficient with sexual excitement (the better to enjoy the body scent of our lover) some people sneeze when they become aroused. Similar changes in the membranes of the nose probably account for the phenomenon known as 'bride's cold'.

The intense pleasure we can derive from the physical act of smelling cannot be overestimated. Ironically, while we are likely to enjoy the secret scents of a loved one in silence, we will often give orgasmic gasps and theatrical impressions of rapture when smelling delicious food, aromatic wine or a perfume-laden flower.

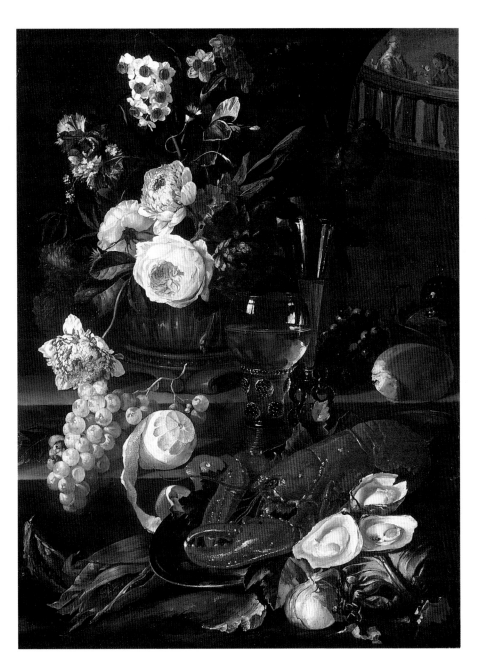

ABOVE: *Still Life*, A.Caproens, nineteenth century
OPPOSITE PAGE: Drawing by Martin van Maele, died 1926

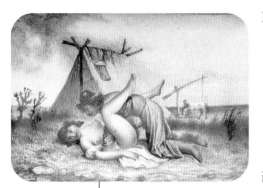

If orgasm is 'la petite mort' (the little death) then sneezing is 'le petit orgasme.' The sensation of sneezing can be so pleasurable and satisfying that the habit of taking snuff became very popular during the eighteenth and nineteenth centuries. Snuff is produced from finely-milled tobacco and can be blended to a wide variety of aromas and strengths. The rather unlikely idea of inhaling aromatic dust which among other things provokes the reflex of sneezing was satirized by Bob Newhart in his imaginary dialogue with Sir Walter Raleigh (1552-1618) who is credited with first bringing tobacco from the New World.

From the beginning, jewellers had produced a variety of snuff boxes both in precious metals and enamel to add to the aesthetic pleasure of snuff taking. In the nineteenth century new technology brought snuff and snuff boxes to the mass market and tins decorated with oleographs became popular. Reflecting the secret erotic connotations of snuff, some of these boxes – particularly those made in France and Russia – contained, as did the pill boxes used by ladies, erotic miniatures.

A selection of eighteenth and nineteenth-century boxes are reproduced here.

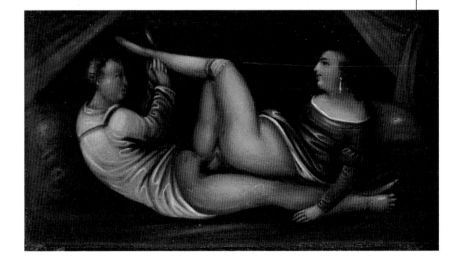

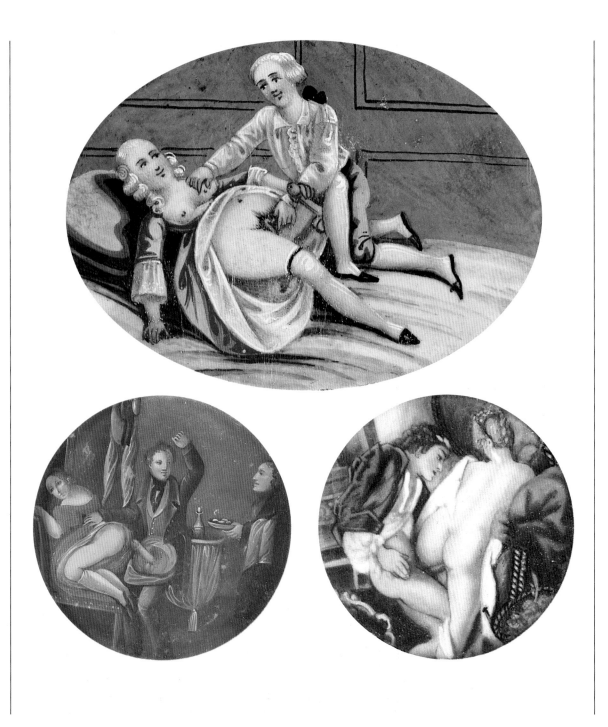

Last night my kisses drowned in the softness of black hair

And my kisses like bees went plundering the softness

of black hair

Last night my hands were thrust in the mystery of black hair,

And my kisses like bees went plundering the sweetness of

pomegranates.

And among the scents of the harvest above my queen's neck the harvest

of black hair

And my teeth played with the golden skin of her two ears.

Last night my kisses drowned in the softness of black hair

And my kisses like bees went plundering the softness of

of black hair.

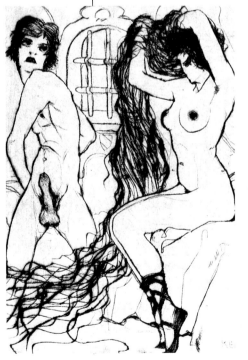

The unknown Afghan poet is eloquent about hair and its impact on our senses. The visual and tactile qualities of hair are dealt with elsewhere, but the way it affects our sense of smell is no less important. Hair both holds and disperses scent: this may be our own body perfume or an aroma we have chosen to add to it. Naturally, in long hair these qualities are accentuated. Literature is full of unforgettable images of hair eroticism and even fetishism, from the fairy tale *Rapunzel* and Guinevere's 'golden hair' in Tennyson's *Idylls of the King*, to Zola's *Nana* and *The Rape of the Lock* by Alexander Pope (1688-1744):

'Fair tresses man's imperial race insnare,

And beauty draws us with a single hair.'

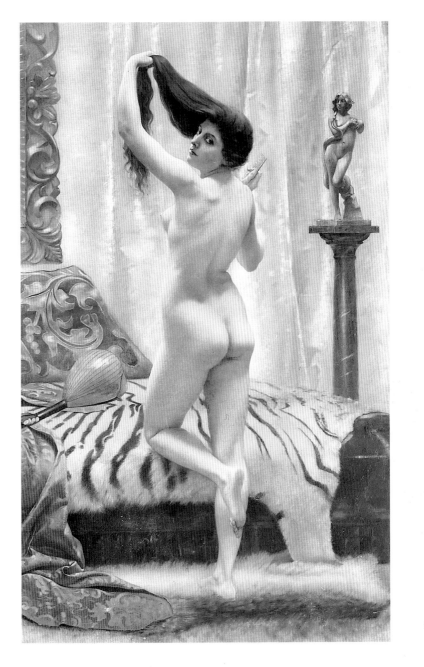

ABOVE: *Before a Mirror*, Robert Barrett Browning, 1846-1912
OPPOSITE PAGE: *Rapunzel*, Rudolf Keller, died 1890

The scent wafted from our head hair like the fumes from an incense burner and diffusing from the whole of our skin surface is transmitting its sexy pheromone message constantly. Augmented by the scent traps of body hair which Nature has thoughtfully provided at the strategic sites of pubis and armpit, our highly personal message is full of erotic suggestion – providing, of course, there is someone out there who wants to receive the olfactory equivalent of an obscene telephone call. And once our message is received, and moves from the unconscious to the conscious mind, how do we actually smell to one another? Women have some inkling of this since they rather like their own intimate scents: it seems appropriate therefore to give both the first and the last word on this to the Shulamite from the *Song of Songs*:

'My beloved is gone down to his gardens, to the beds of spices
To feed in the gardens, and to gather lilies.
I am my beloved's and my beloved is mine:
He feedeth his flock among the lilies.'

In his *Mémoires* Casanova wrote: 'There is something in the air of the bedroom of the woman one loves, something so intimate, so balsamic, such voluptuous emanations, that if a lover had to choose between Heaven and this place of delight his hesitation would not last for a moment.' In his very different *Private Memoirs*, Sir Kenelm Digby finds his lover asleep: 'on her breasts did glisten a few drops of sweatlike diamond sparks, and had a more fragrant odour than the violets or primroses whose season was newly passed.'

In Tolstoy's *War and Peace* Count Peter decides to marry Princess Helena after inhaling her intimate odour at a ball. Huysmans (1848-1907) whose novels reek of every kind of perfume and who disliked balls because their olfactory impact was too powerful, wrote what amounts to an elegy to the armpit:

'Various as the colour of the hair, the odour of the armpit is infinitely divisible; its gamut covers the whole keyboard of odours, reaching the obstinate scents of syringa and elder, and sometimes recalling the sweet perfume of the rubbed fingers that have held a cigarette. Audacious and sometimes fatiguing in the brunette and black-haired woman, sharp and fierce in the red-haired woman, the armpit is as heady as some sugared wines in the blondes.'

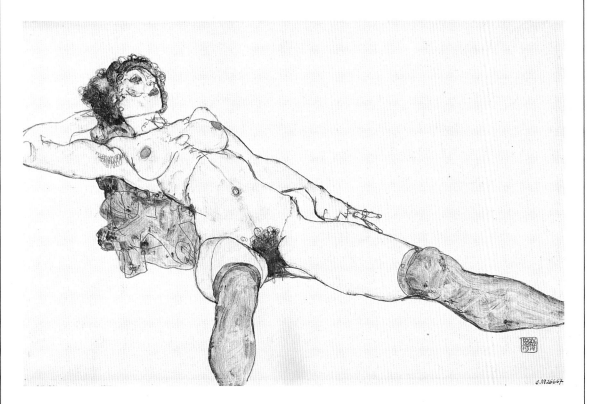

ABOVE: *Reclining nude,* Egon Schiele, 1890-1918

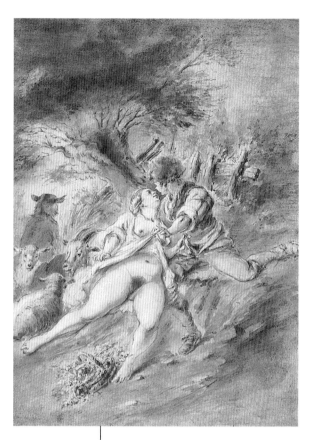

Women describing the scent of men use strongly contrasting metaphors. First is the persuasive voice of Helen Keller (1880-1968) who was both deaf and blind:

'Masculine exhalations are, as a rule, stronger, more vivid, more widely differentiated than those of women. In the odour of young men there is something elemental, as of fire, storm, and salt sea.'

One of the mistresses of H.G.Wells (1866-1946) interrogated by an inquisitive Somerset Maugham (1874-1965) to discover the secret of his success with women, replied: 'his body smells of honey.' Another similarly gentle metaphor appears in the Irish saga Cuchulain of Muirthemne where a woman describes the smell of a group of young men: 'It was the same as if I was in a sweet apple garden'.

In *Faust*, three women discuss Paris:

First: 'Mixed with the incense-steam what odour precious
            steals to my bosom, and my heart refreshes?'

Second: 'Forsooth, it penetrates and warms the feeling!
            It comes from him.'

Third: 'His flower of youth, unsealing,
            It is: Youth's fine ambrosia, ripe, unfading,
            The atmosphere around his form pervading.'

Finally, the Shulamite in the *Song of Songs* sings of her bridegroom:

'My beloved is unto me as a bundle of myrrh,

That lieth between my breasts.

My beloved is unto me as a cluster of henna-flowers

In the vineyards of En-gedi.'

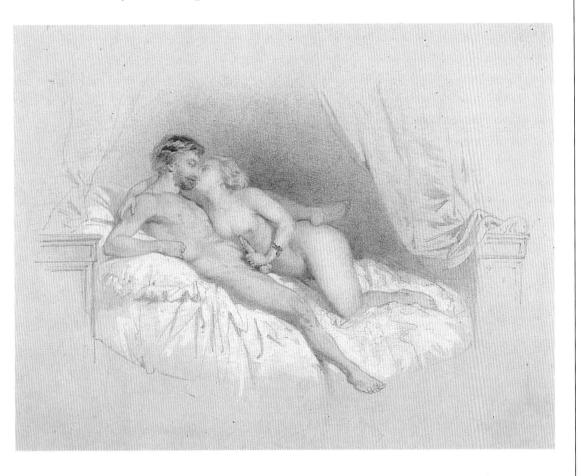

ABOVE: *Lovers,* Edouard de Beaumont, 1821-1888
OPPOSITE PAGE: *Lover's Hour,* after Jean-Baptiste Marie Huet, 1745-1811

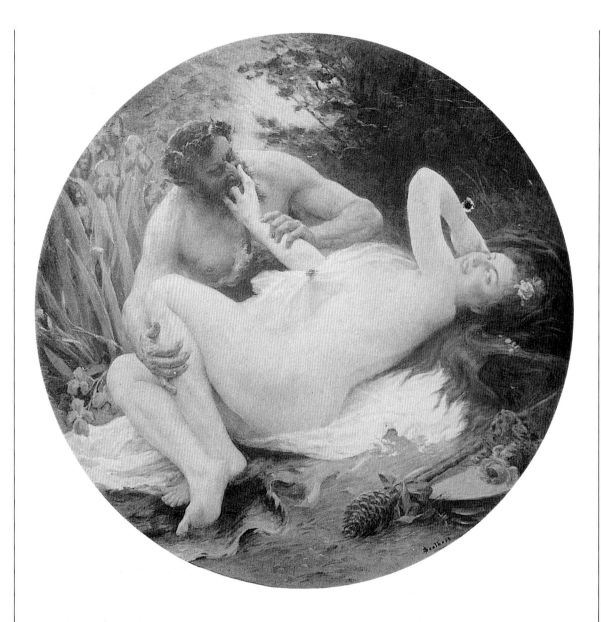

OPPOSITE PAGE: Anonymous watercolour, Napoleonic period
ABOVE: *Pan with a Nymph*, coloured lithograph, nineteenth century

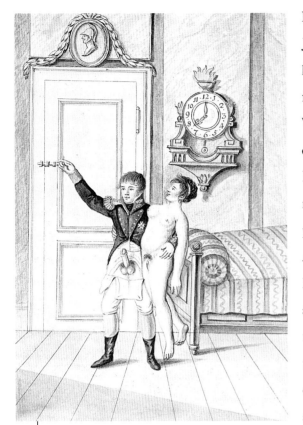

Napoleon, in a famous letter to the Empress Josephine, asked her 'not to wash' while awaiting his return, implying clearly that he wished their first embraces to be an olfactory banquet. Whether he intended to wash was never made clear. But in another celebrated comment the Emperor seems to contradict himself when he rhapsodizes about the courtesan he had been provided with somewhere between Ulm and Austerlitz: 'one of the most agreeable women I have ever known – no smell at all!' We are ambiguous about odour. Perhaps Casanova gives us a clue to why that should be so in the preface to his *Mémoires:* 'I have always found sweet the odour of the women I have loved.' Perhaps love – as in so many things – is the key. Where love is not a factor we had better pay particular attention to our toilet, since our personal scent can either inflame passion, or inundate it. The Emperor's bedfellow for a night was taking no chances.

The human body, washed regularly and thoroughly, has quite enough natural odour. Anything less than scrupulous hygiene, particularly in the obvious scent traps, is a more effective way of killing passion than a cold shower unless we are anosmic, or emperors. The Roman poet Ovid (43BC - 17AD) in his *Art of Love* sums all this up in one succinct line: Ne trux caper iret in alas, 'do not keep a goat in your armpit'.

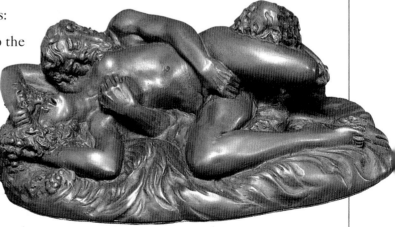

At about the time that the exiled Ovid was writing his *Art of Love* and making jokes about goats and armpits, a mysterious voice echoed over the Ionian Sea announcing that 'the great god Pan is dead!' The emperor Tiberius – a perfect example of absolute power corrupting absolutely – believed this, which says something for his mental state at the beginning of his long decline into debauchery.

Pan, half man and half goat, epitomizes our dual nature: the animal and the civilized, the physical and the cerebral. Images of Pan – and his followers, the satyrs or fauns – occur throughout Western art from the Classical period onwards. It was a convenient way of depicting explicit sexuality since that is what Pan and his satyrs did most of the time with the accommodating nymphs (hence nymphomania and satyriasis). But images of Pan are more than erotic art, they are a useful reminder that our bodies are animal, with animal needs and animal senses. Of course we have brains and higher feelings as well as bodies: the essence of civilization is to keep the two in balance. If we deny our normal healthy instincts we do so at our peril; if we forget to enjoy all our senses to the full, we are doomed to have all the inconvenience of a body with few of its benefits.

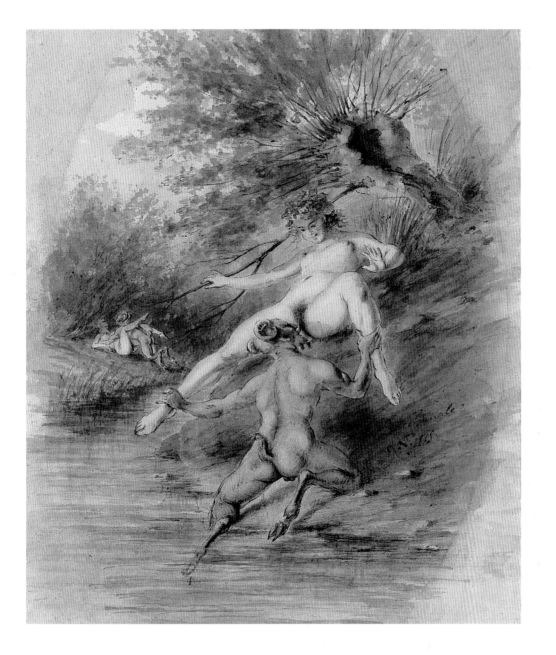

ABOVE: French watercolour, anonymous, 1815
OPPOSITE PAGE, TOP: Fragment of an Attic bowl, circa 500 BC
OPPOSITE PAGE, BOTTOM: *Nymph and Satyr*, bronze, nineteenth century

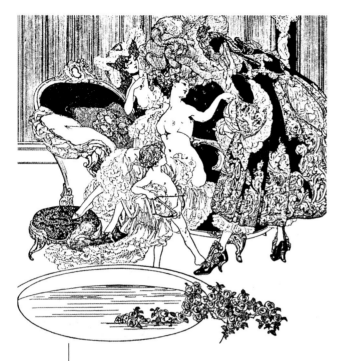

The rituals of bathing can be pleasurable. Whenever possible the necessity of keeping our personal scent at civilized rather than wildlife levels should not be a rushed affair, but slow, relaxing and sensual. The Romans recognized that baths are one of the keystones of civilization: they built them everywhere they went, from the cold north of England to Palestine, from southern Spain to the Black Sea. Our more modest baths can be just as enjoyable if we have the right attitude. The bathroom can be a peaceful cell to which we retire like sensual Trappists, contemplating our

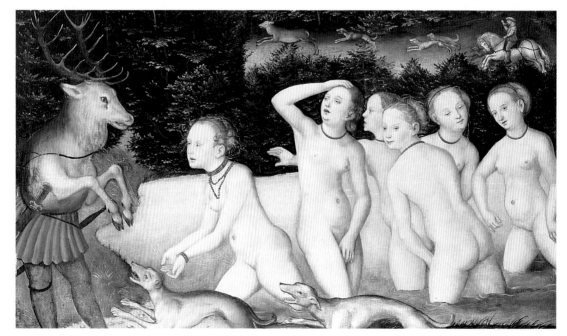

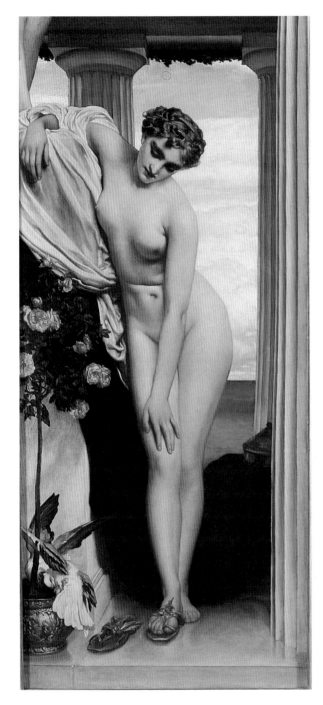

navels through the steam. Or bathing can be noisy, shared and altogether steamier. If we are as close to our lover as we should be, solitary bathing is probably to be preferred, with sharing as an occasional treat. Always make sure you are invited! When the goddess Diana received an unscheduled visit from Actaeon while bathing, his punishment was to be turned into a stag and hunted by his own hounds.

LEFT: *Venus Disrobing for the Bath*, Lord Leighton, 1830-1896

OPPOSITE PAGE, BOTTOM: *Diana and Actaeon*, Lucas Cranach, 1472-1553
OPPOSITE PAGE, TOP: Drawing by Franz von Bayros

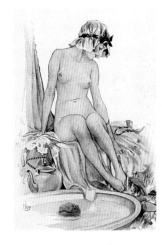

The erotic and auto-erotic possibilities of bathing are explored in this extract from *The Voluptuous Confessions of a French Lady of Fashion*, first published in the Victorian magazine *The Boudoir*:

'There was in the pavilion a chamber pot and wash basin; I saw Bertha fill the latter, lift up her petticoats, and stoop over it. She was placed right in front of me, and nothing could escape my view. As she did this her slit opened, it seemed to me a much more lively carnation; the interior and the edges, even up to the fleecy mound which surrounded it, seemed inundated with the same liquor which I had seen come from Monsieur B.

'Bertha commenced an ample ablution... all at once I saw her stop still, then a finger fixed upon a little eminence which showed itself prominently; this finger rubbed lightly at first, then with a kind of fury. At length Bertha gave the same symptoms of pleasure which I had often seen before.'

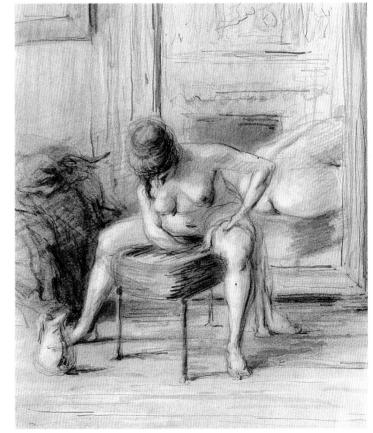

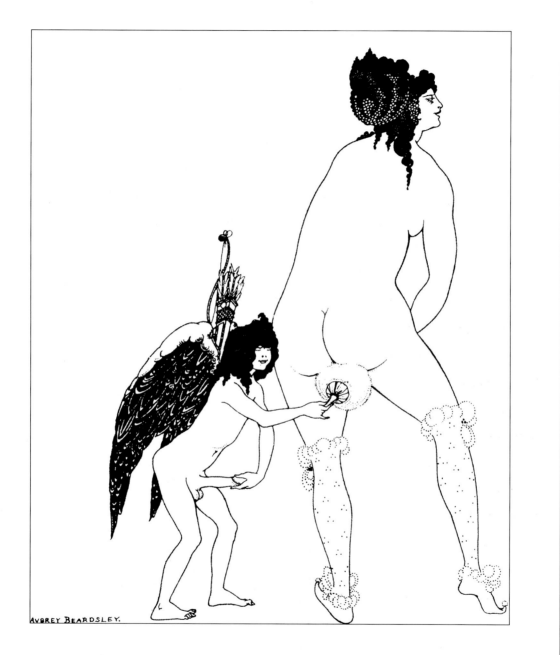

AUBREY BEARDSLEY.

ABOVE: *The Toilet of Lampito,* from Lysistrata, Aubrey Beardsley
OPPOSITE PAGE, BOTTOM: *The Bidet,* Jean Louis Forain, 1852-1931
OPPOSITE PAGE, TOP: Postcard, 1920

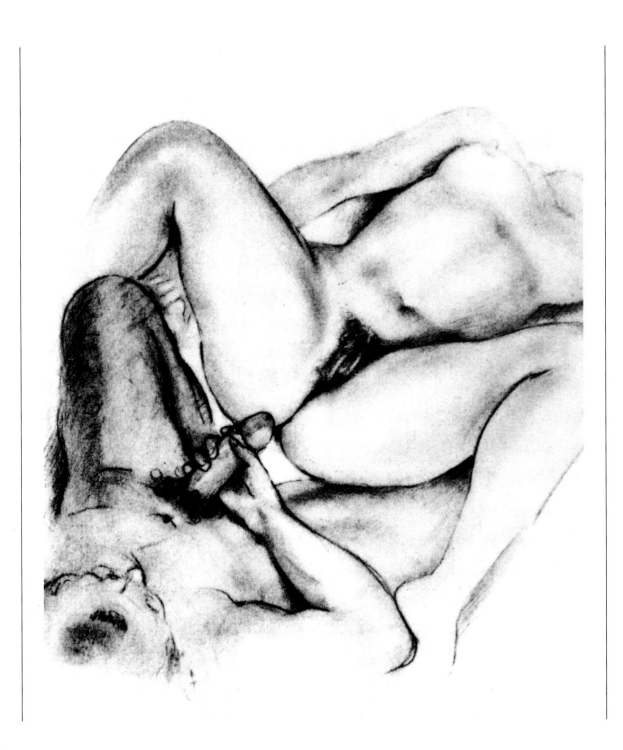

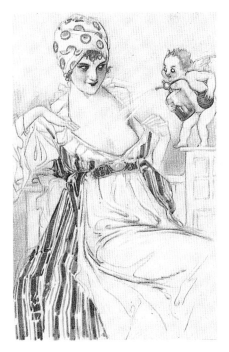

Bathing – accompanied or unaccompanied – is made much more sensual if we borrow scents from nature to add to the hot water. These essences range from the astringency of limes and the spartan delights of pine forests, to spicy sandalwood and the warm femininity of rose bulgar.

So many bath perfumes are now available and in so many combinations as soaps, essence, salts, milks, oils – or as individual essential oils we can mix ourselves – that we are embarrassed for choice. The rule, as for your main perfume, is to find something you like and which complements your own natural perfume.

In *Kama Sutra*, Vatsyayana makes much of the sensual pleasures of 'shampooing', a cross between massage and washing. Bathing and soaping one another is our modern equivalent of shampooing. It may lead to lovemaking or it may not: it is pleasant and tender in either case.

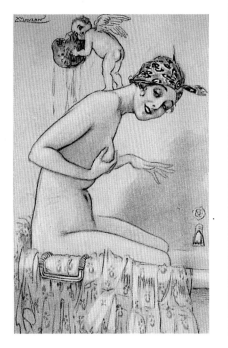

TOP AND BOTTOM: French postcards, 1920
OPPOSITE PAGE: Drawing by an unknown artist, circa 1930

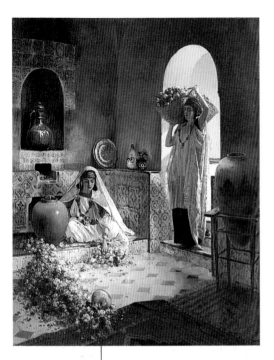

The scent of rain on warm earth reminds

me darling of your sweet breath. And those small winds that

uncurl the deodar flowers petal by petal

and drenched in that heady sap blow south,

I grasp, embrace, pretending it's you.

But darling, my excuse,

if any ask why I'm making a fool of myself

making love to thin air,

is that no breeze could be so fragrant

had it not first caressed your body.

From *The Cloud Messenger* by Kalidasa (5th century AD)

Perfume is uniquely personal to an individual because each carefully prepared blend, whether simple or complex, combines with and 'exalts' the body's natural scent. Perfume's origins are less subtle. Until comparatively recently the skills of the perfumer were not pleasantly combined with those of the plumber, so much as intended to replace them.

You say y'are sweet; how sh'd we know

Whether that you be sweet or no?

From powders and perfumes keep free;

Then we shall smell how sweet you be.

On a Perfum'd Lady, Robert Herrick

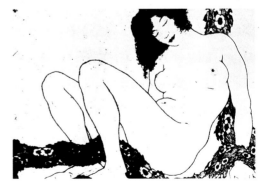

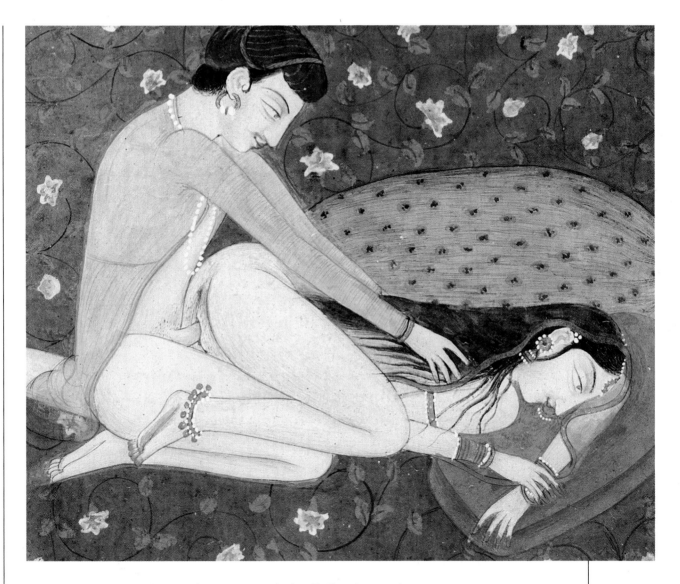

ABOVE: Anonymous painting, India, nineteenth century
OPPOSITE PAGE, TOP: *The Rose Gatherers,* Rudolph Ernst, 1854-1920
OPPOSITE PAGE, BOTTOM: Pen drawing, M.E.Phillipp, Germany circa 1912

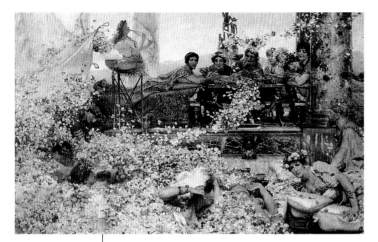

The choosing of a perfume must always be a personal matter. When you find one which suits you stay with it. Change your soaps and bath essences if you must, but stay with your main perfume until your entire wardrobe is tinged with it, until it becomes an adjunct of your personality, until people who know you detect it on another but still say that it is your perfume. Those who change perfumes with their clothes completely miss the point. At best the olfactory impression they make is confused and easily forgotten, like faces dimly remembered at a party. At worst it is jarring.

Women generally have a better sense of smell than men which, like all gifts, is both a blessing and a curse. But it means that they are more capable of remembering their lover's own smell and enjoying it, in a society where men use perfume less.

None of our senses has the ability to unlock the gates of memory which the sense of smell has. The aroma of the most mundane things – carbolic soap, bonfires, seaweed, different things for different people – has the power to take us on a journey in time and space back to our childhood.

Helen Keller called smell the 'fallen angel'. Certainly it has no time for conventional morality. A woman who knows how to use perfume will be with her lover again each time he smells it, wherever he is, whoever he is with, until the day he dies.

ABOVE: *Roses of Heliogabalus,* Sir Lawrence Alma-Tadema, 1836-1912
OPPOSITE PAGE: *The Heart of the Rose,* Sir Edward Burne-Jones, 1833-1898

Last night, ah, yesternight, betwixt her lips and mine

There fell thy shadow, Cynara! thy breath was shed

Upon my soul between the kisses and the wine;

And I was desolate and sick of an old passion,

Yea I was desolate and bowed my head:

I have been faithful to thee, Cynara! in my fashion.

I have forgot much, Cynara! gone with the wind,

Flung roses, roses riotously with the throng,

Dancing, to put thy pale, lost lilies out of mind;

But I was desolate and sick of an old passion

Yea, all the time, because the dance was long:

I have been faithful to thee, Cynara! in my fashion.

Ernest Dowson (1867-1900)

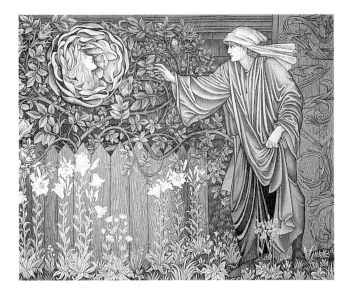

There is a kind of science-fiction logic to the fact that flowers develop their maximum fragrance when they are sexually receptive in order to attract insects to pollinate them, and we harvest (or replicate) those fragrances and blend them into aphrodisiacs. There is no question that most perfume is intended to be aphrodisiac in its effect.

The exceptions to this are the 'male' after-shave preparations such as Eau-de-Cologne, Hungarian Water, Lavender Water and all the sharp children they have fostered. The same can be said of mouthwashes, deodorants and other preparations containing menthol, eucalyptus oil, peppermint oil and camphor, which is used in racing stables to quieten down mares in heat. Interestingly, the smell of horse urine was once thought to have (and may indeed have) an aphrodisiac effect on humans. A bizarre fact which gives us a clue to the elements which occur in all the more successful erotic perfumes.

Having plundered the vegetable kingdom for sexual stimulants, the perfumers turned their attention to an unsuspecting animal world. Amber, civet and musk have been used in incense and perfume for millennia. Amber has a smell similar to human head and genital aroma, and was even ingested as an aphrodisiac in the Middle Ages. Civet, from the Arabic for 'froth', is reminiscent of cat's urine and faeces. Musk, from the Sanskrit for 'testicle' and itself a sexual secretion, is strongly reminiscent of intimate human body odours. These fugitives from a witch's cauldron are still used today by the great perfume houses, an essential ingredient in perfumes we would all recognize.

We have come across 'musk' before, in muscat wine. Its unmistakable odour occurs throughout nature in both plants and animals. Eastern love poetry is full of 'musk' similes: 'her navel is filled with musk' (Persia); 'and on the breeze, the perfume of your musky nest' (China).

Musk – redolent with human urine and vaginal secretions – and the capryl group of odours – pungent with armpit aroma and equally widespread in nature – are essential elements in many of the most sensuous and erotic perfumes. How can this be? The great god Pan rears his horned head again (caprylic acid is after all from the Latin 'caper' meaning goat) reminding us that eroticism – in everything – is a balance between the animal and the civilized.

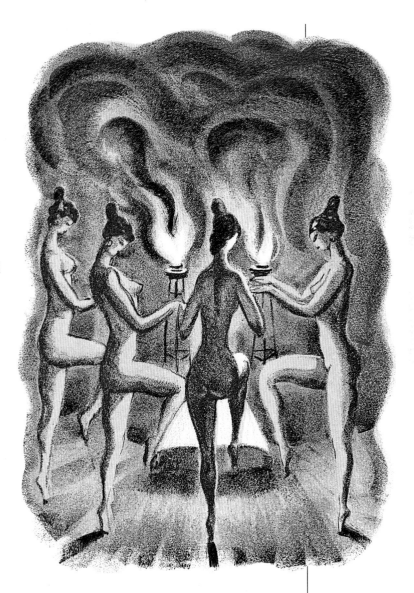

OPPOSITE PAGE: Drawing by 'A1', Vienna, 1935
ABOVE: Coloured lithograph, André Provot

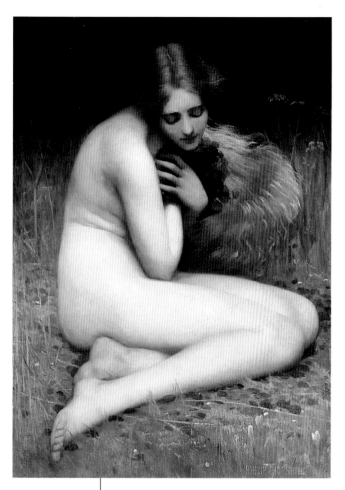

The alchemy of perfume begins with flowers. To smell a rose is erotic. To smell rose perfume on a woman is erotic. No doubt Mark Antony found the rose perfume wafting from the sails of Cleopatra's famous barge and intended to announce her imminent arrival, highly erotic. But on the 'palette' of a master perfumer, rose has a 'colour' described as narcotic. Violets, too, are narcotic rather than erotic, yet this was the perfume of the Empress Josephine, a highly sensual and sexual woman. Napoleon planted violets on her grave and wore them in a locket for the rest of his life. Do the narcotic aromas prepare our senses for the woman's own scent, is that the secret? Perfumery is more like magic than science.

Some flowers, especially white ones, make erotic statements of their own. Lilies, in marked contrast to their chaste image, have a sultry aroma. Vatsyayana describes the sex of the beautiful Padmini woman as 'perfumed like the lily that has newly burst.' Chestnut and whitethorn have a strong feminine odour as does the wild *Chenopodium vulvaria*, called 'erba connina' in Italy, 'conio' in Normandy and – which would please Pan – 'stinking goatsfoot' in England.

In sexual surveys a simile frequently used to describe the smell of semen is 'flowering grasses' or 'crushed grass'. Havelock Ellis (1859-1939) in his monumental *Studies in the Psychology of Sex* attributes 'a very decided spermatic odour' to henna flowers . An idea which sheds new light on the extract from the *Song of Songs* quoted on page 103!

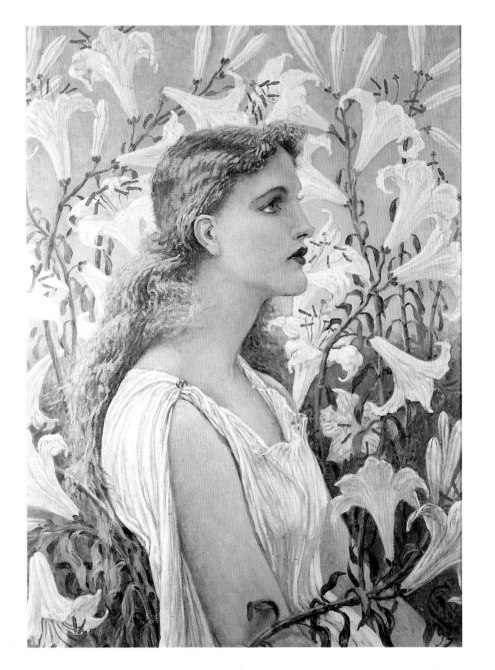

ABOVE: *Lilies*, Walter Crane, 1845-1915
OPPOSITE PAGE: *Wood Nymph*, Phillip J. Thornhill, circa 1900

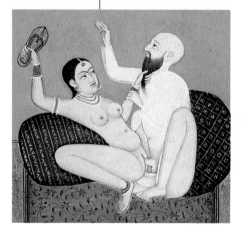

Were he to appear in any main street in the Western world today, where every third shop seems to be selling shoes, Restif de la Bretonne (1734-1806) would – if he is not already there – assume he had gone to heaven. Because the 'Voltaire of the chambermaids' and the 'Rousseau of the gutter' was literature's most notorious shoe fetishist. He was not, however, the only person in literature who derived erotic pleasure from shoes – and feet, because as Restif says 'the factitious taste for the shoe is only a reflection of that for pretty feet'.

Ovid never tires of writing about the erotic joys of feet; Goethe's *Wahlverwandschaften* contains a description of the foot's beauty and the delights of kissing the shoe of a lover, nor are the erotic possibilities of feet lost on the cobbler in Thomas Hardy's *Under the Greenwood Tree. Cinderella*, in common with many fairy tales, involves some very obvious sexual symbolism as does the less well-known story of *Rhodope*. This famous courtesan had her sandal stolen by an eagle who dropped it into the king's lap. Naturally he fell in love with the shoe's owner and did not rest until he made her his queen.

All this erotic excitement is mainly because of odour. It is true that the shoe is also a symbol of the female genitals, and that stiletto heels and buckles are much in demand among sado-masochists, but in general the erotic interest in feet and shoes is driven by the sense of smell. The aroma of leather is also sexually exciting to many people. In a society with so many shrines to the Foot in its high streets, it is difficult to regard all this as anything other than normal. The last fevered word on the subject comes from an expert, Restif de la Bretonne, who wanted to be buried with the slipper of Colette Parangon, the love of his life:

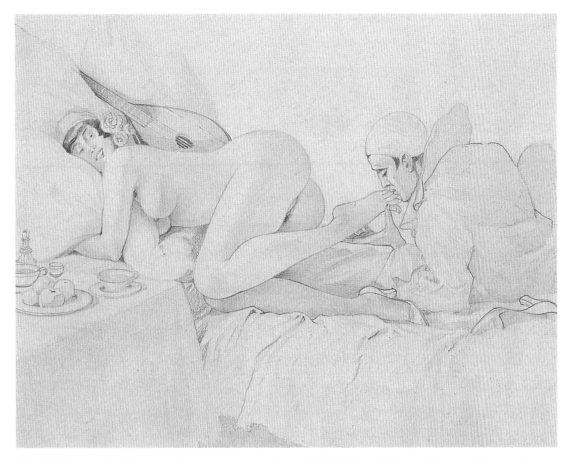

'Carried away by the most impetuous passion and idolizing Colette, I seemed to see her and touch her in handling what she had just worn (rose-coloured shoes); my lips pressed one of these jewels while the other, deceiving the sacred end of nature, from excess of exaltation replaced the object of sex (I cannot express myself more clearly). The warmth which she had communicated to the insensible object which had touched her still remained and gave a soul to it; a voluptuous cloud covered my eyes.'

ABOVE: *The Beautiful Foot,* Franz Kuna, died 1881
OPPOSITE PAGE, TOP: Postcard, France, circa 1925
OPPOSITE PAGE, BOTTOM: Indian miniature, Rajasthan, eighteenth century

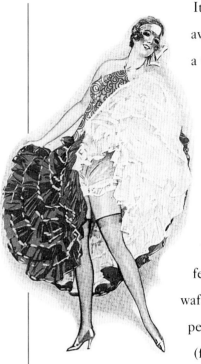

It is clear from his writing that Goethe (1749-1832) was very aware of odour and its sexual importance. He records that to make a two-day absence from Weimar and Frau von Stein more bearable, he took with him a bodice she had been wearing so that he could inhale the perfume of her body. This is not fetishism – except in the crudest sense – it is love.

The odour-absorbing properties of clothes, and the erotic possibilities these create, do not have to be sanctified by love. The absinthe drinkers in the Moulin Rouge enjoyed not only the spectacle and music of the can-can, but an erotic barrage of feminine scents wafted from shaken petticoats. In Sevillana (flamenco) the sinuous intertwining, with arms raised, together with the abrupt skirt flapping is not only designed to excite the eye. Nor is the fan simply a fashion accessory: it disperses the skin's perfume as well as cooling its surface.

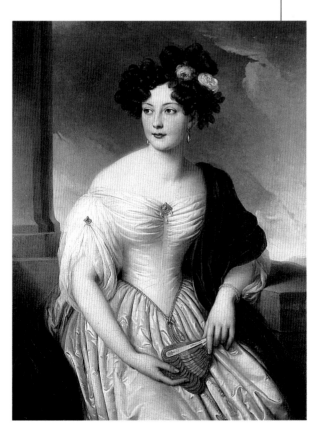

Huysmans, high priest of the sense of smell, regarded clothes as the ultimate refinement of olfactory sensuality, the different layers and materials orchestrating the erotic impact. Two centuries earlier Robert Herrick wrote a poem with much the same idea.

Tell, if thou canst, and truly, whence did come

This camphire, storax, spikenard, galbanum:

These musks, these ambers, and these other smells,

Sweet as the vestrie of the oracles.

Ile tell thee; while my Julia did unlace

Her silken bodies, but a breathing space...

from *Upon Julia's Unlacing Herself*

OPPOSITE PAGE, TOP: Advertisement for the Moulin Rouge
OPPOSITE PAGE, BOTTOM: *Lady with a Fan,* Johann Ender, 1793-1854

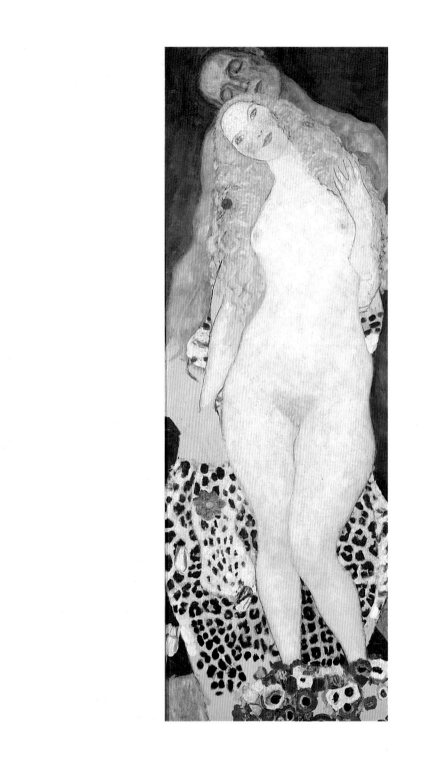

HEARING

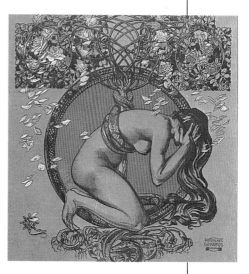

Hearing is the sense which binds the other senses together in harmony. It is also the sense most concerned with interaction between human beings: it is the foundation of language, which is communication between minds, and music which is the communication between hearts

Helen Keller, who could neither see nor hear, regarded her deafness as a '... worse misfortune. For it means the loss of the most vital stimulus – the sound of the voice that brings language, sets thoughts astir and keeps us in the intellectual company of man.'

The voice has immense power. This lies not only in what is said or the language in which it is expressed, but in its timbre . The Fall of Man would never have occurred if the serpent in the Garden of Eden had spoken with the hissing sibilants of a nursery python. We can be quite sure that the voice of temptation was a resonant baritone, thrilling Eve's senses with its sound, her imagination with its words.

OPPOSITE PAGE: *Adam and Eva* (unfinished), Gustav Klimt, 1917/18
Above: Art Nouveau poster, Giovanni Mataloni, circa 1900

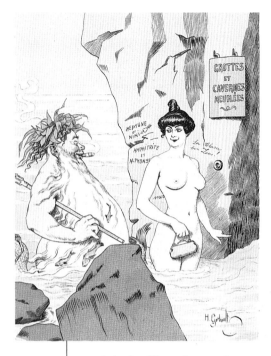

The erotic power of the voice, particularly when singing and accompanied by music, is epitomized in the myth of the Sirens who lured sailors to their death. The Lorelei who haunts the rock on the Rhine near St Goar, celebrated in the poem by Heinrich Heine (1797-1856), and the numerous mermaid legends, are variations on the same theme. In the Greek myth, crafty Odysseus – warned by another enchantress, his lover the nymph Circe – cheats the Sirens by having himself tied to the mast of his ship as it passes Sicily, while his companions stop their ears with wax. But what sound could be so enticing, so sexually charged that it is stronger even than the will to self-preservation? Do we begin to understand what it might be like when a singer moves us physically and makes our flesh tingle? When another Greek in Italy, the young Maria Callas (1923-1977), put all the dramatic power of her incomparable voice into the slightly unsuitable part of Puccini's *Madame Butterfly* and brought the whole cynical La Scala audience to its feet, was that an echo of the Sirens?

In some versions of the Siren myth, the sea nymphs imitate the voices of loved ones. That would indeed be potent auditory magic. Our response to the unique combination of tone, pitch and rhythm which is the voice of someone we love is so strong that the telephone can almost be regarded as a sexual aid during periods of separation.

OPPOSITE PAGE: *The Cave of the Storm Nymphs,* Sir Edward Poynter, 1836-1919
ABOVE: *La Sirène,* H.Gerbault

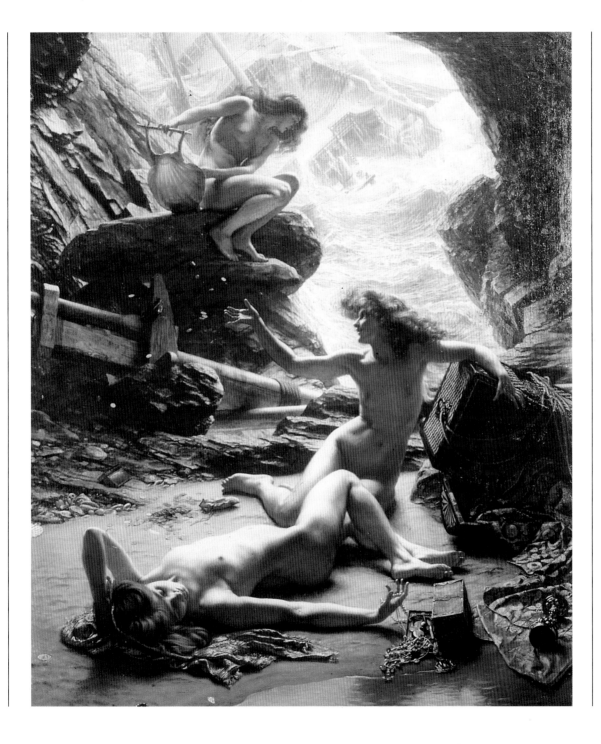

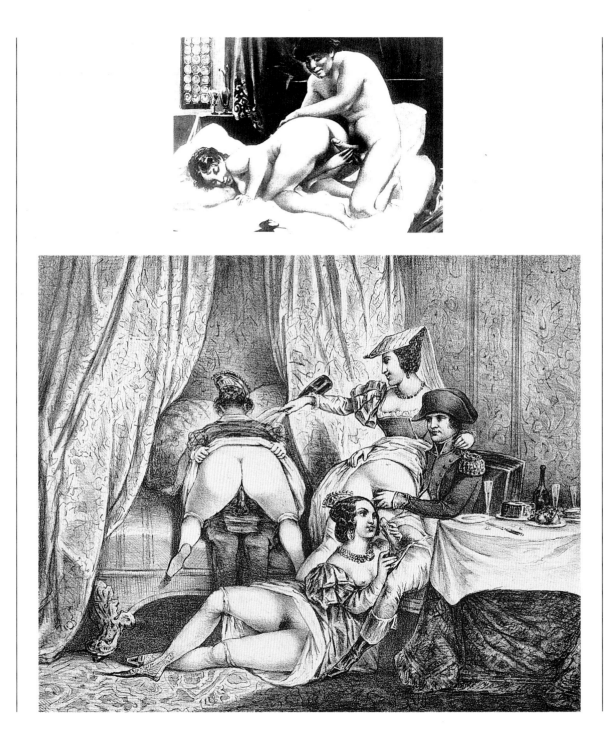

The reciprocal sounds of lovemaking – either physical, inarticulate or urgently articulate – are an essential part of the sexual drama. This fiercely erotic auditory extract is from the pastiche novel *Memoirs of a Venetian Courtesan:*

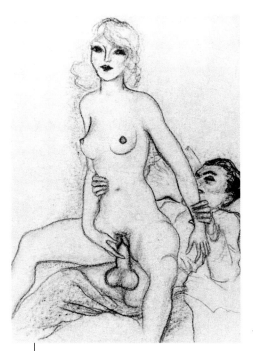

'I turned my back to him and knelt on the bed, legs apart. Burying my face deep down in the soft mattress, haunches raised, I offered myself to him. Marco knelt in his turn, but on the floor, and gently opened the lips of my sex. His tongue lapped urgently in the moist portal... Then its tip became a point. I felt it searching... around my lips, on the swollen bud of my clitoris. I moaned for him to put his cock in me.

'He stook up behind me and slowly pushed... into me right up to the hilt. Just as slowly he withdrew, pulling right out, then in again opening the soft folds of my sex. Slowly, again and again, until the moist suction of each pulling-out and pushing-in itself made the sound Fu'ck! Fu'ck!'

Salvador Dali (1904 -1989) told the story that when he was young and sexually inexperienced he suffered a period of temporary impotence because he had read in an erotic novel that a woman who is made love to from the back makes the sound of breaking open a ripe watermelon. Dali became obsessed with the exciting idea, and increasingly certain that he could never reproduce such a luscious sound. It ended well, but inflammatory prose – erotic or otherwise – should never be taken too seriously.

ABOVE: Pencil drawing by 'Al' Vienna, 1935
OPPOSITE PAGE, BOTTOM: *Bonaparte en Italie*, lithograph, France, circa 1830
OPPOSITE PAGE, TOP: Heliogravure, anonymous, 1892

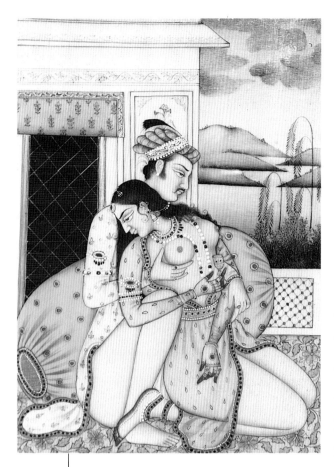

'Her first shy cries may sound to you like sobbing doves, the cuckoo's call climbing in the leaves, woodpigeon's drowsy sighing, the shrill shriek of her parrot in its cage. But soon your lady, moaning like a black bee, piping like a startled moorhen, uttering low harsh cries that sound like wild geese and wild ducks calling on the wing, ends yammering shameless as a quail.'

from *Kama Sutra*

After describing the inarticulate sounds women make when making love, Mallanaga Vatsyayana adds wisely: 'About these things there cannot be either enumeration or any definite rule. Congress having once commenced, passion alone gives birth to all the acts of the parties.' Vatsyayana says nothing of the male part in what should, after all, be a duet. But women do tend to be more vocal than men in their lovemaking. This beautiful extract is from *Lady Chatterley's Lover:*

'When awareness of the outside began to come back, she clung to his breast, murmuring 'My love! My love!' And he held her silently. And she curled on his breast, perfect.

But his silence was fathomless. His hands held her like flowers, so still and strange. 'Where are you?' she whispered to him. 'Where are you? Speak to me! Say something to me!'

He kissed her softly, murmuring: 'Ay, my lass!' But she did not know what he meant, she did not know where he was. In his silence he seemed lost to her.

'You love me, don't you?' she murmured.

'Ay, tha knows!' he said.

'But tell me!' she pleaded.

'Ay! Ay! 'asn't ter felt it?' he said dimly, but softly and surely. And she clung close to him, closer. He was so much more peaceful in love than she was, and she wanted him to reassure her.'

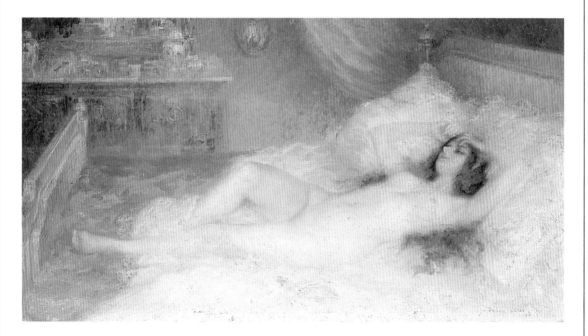

OPPOSITE PAGE: *Padmini woman*, Rajasthan,
ABOVE: *Nude,* Pierre Franc-Lamy, 1855-1919

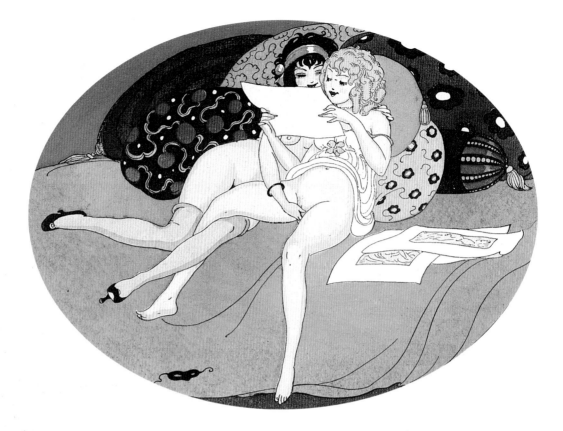

The taboo 'four-letter' words in *Lady Chatterley's Lover* for which D.H.Lawrence was vilified are more or less commonplace today, not in the bedroom or talking of the bedroom where they should be, but as expletives – the very thing Lawrence hated. He said of his last book, which was to have been called *Tenderness:* 'I want men and women to be able to think sex, fully, completely, honestly and clearly… I always labour at the same thing, to make the sex relation valid and precious, instead of shameful.' W.B.Yeats (1865-1939) said of *Lady Chatterley's Lover:* 'the coarse language of the one, accepted by both, becomes a forlorn poetry uniting their solitudes, something ancient, humble and terrible.'

The value of the words 'fuck' and 'cunt' is that they are the very best words in the English language for what they describe . This remains true despite the fact that we misuse the words and the power in them because we are too lazy to use a full vocabulary.

Lawrence's contemporary Lytton Strachey (1880-1932) wrote a sexual satire to amuse his friends. Among other things, *Ermyntrude and Esmeralda*, an imaginary correspondence between two upper-class English girls, points out the absurdity of sexual euphemism:

'I was very excited to see what his bow-wow was like, but I was astonished to see that he hadn't got one, but a very funny big pink thing standing straight up instead. I was rather frightened, because I thought he might be deformed, which wouldn't have been at all nice, so I asked him what it was. Then he laughed so much that I thought everyone would hear, and at last I discovered that it was his bow-wow after all, and it turns out that that is what they get like when they pout! I was very pleased indeed, and so was my pussy when his bow-wow went into it, and after that we went to bed.'

OPPOSITE PAGE: Coloured engraving, France, 1917
ABOVE: Drawing, Franz von Bayros

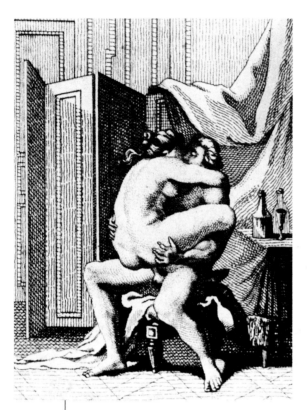

The plain language of love, even when used in the right way, is not always pure in intention. John Wilmot, the second Earl of Rochester (1647-1680), lived the life of debauchery which many aristocrats, past and present, have pursued. But Rochester, a favourite of Charles the Second, had the intellect and wit to satirize his own spectacular dissolution and that of his fellow revellers in the danse macabre of the Restoration Court. In this extract from *The Imperfect Enjoyment*, his poem about premature ejaculation ('A touch from any part of her had done't: Her hand, her foot, her very look's a cunt') and subsequent impotence, Rochester berates his recalcitrant penis:

Worst part of me, and henceforth hated most,

Through all the town a common fucking post,

On whom each whore relieves her tingling cunt

As hogs on gates do rub themselves and grunt,

May'st thou to ravenous chancres be a prey,

Or in consuming weepings waste away;

May strangury and stone thy days attend;

May'st thou ne'er piss, who didst refuse to spend

When all my joys did on false thee depend.

And may ten thousand abler pricks agree

To do the wronged Corinna right for thee.

A world and three centuries away, but united by a common bawdy language, are these lines from *Shave 'em Dry,* a song written and performed by the Twenties blues singer Lucille Bogan. Here the use of four-letter words is celebratory, as vital and raucous as a New Orleans whorehouse:

> A big sow gets fat from eatin corn
> And a pig gets fat from sucking.
> You see this whore, fat like I am?
> Great god I got fat from fuckin!
> My back is made from whalebone,
> And my cock is made of brass,
> And my fuckin is made for workin men
> Who'll go round to kiss my ass!

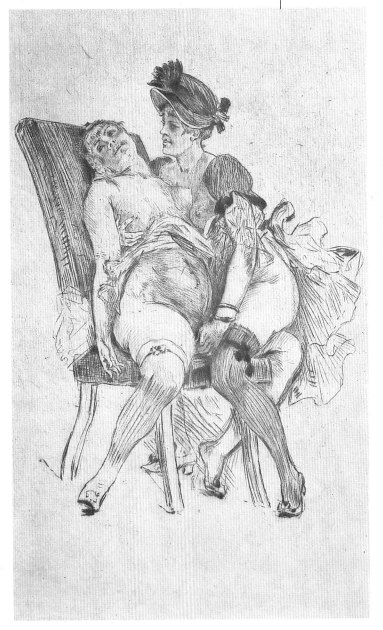

RIGHT: *The Visit,* Félicien Rops,
1835-1898
OPPOSITE PAGE: Anonymous engraving,
eighteenth century

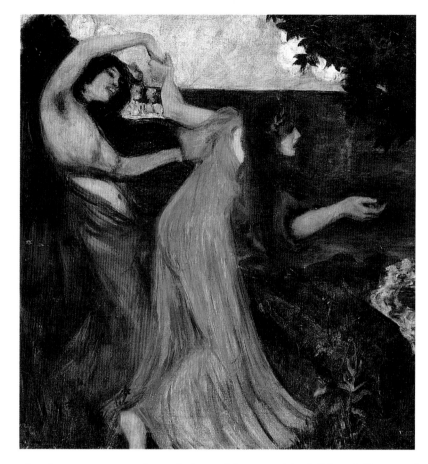

The connection between sex and music is as old as mankind. The ability music has to thrill and move us, its insistent rhythms and satisfying climaxes, are all profoundly erotic. This is equally true of sacred and profane music which – in the distant past when we worshipped gods who embodied the fertility of the earth and of ourselves – were one and the same. The rites of Dionysus, of Osiris and a hundred other gods; the Bacchanalian orgies – all involved music.

Dance, when we give our bodies to the rhythms and spirit of music, has the same origins. Siva, the Hindu god of Creation and Destruction, is also called Lord of the Dance after the moment when his wild rhythms will bring about the end of time itself, just as

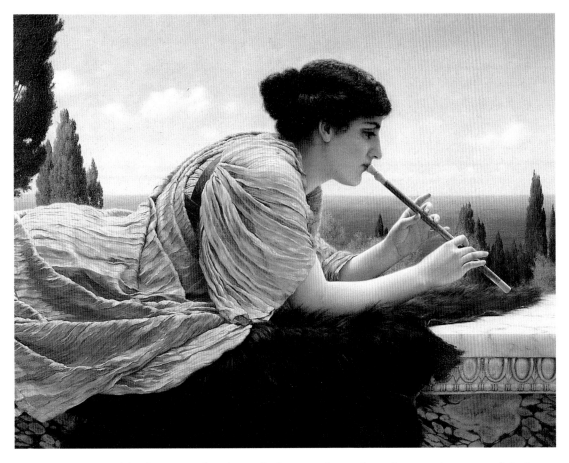

they once created it. Our own dancing mimics creation, often the creative potential of our own bodies in the symbolic sex of the tango or the waltz, or the hearty ritualized orgy of a barn dance.

ABOVE: *The Melody*, John William Godward, 1861-1922
OPPOSITE PAGE: *Calypso*, Andreas Roegels, 1870-1917

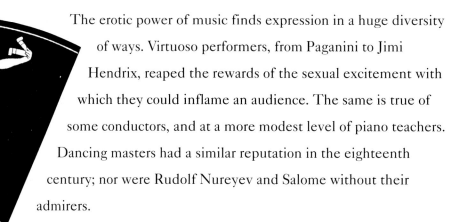

The erotic power of music finds expression in a huge diversity of ways. Virtuoso performers, from Paganini to Jimi Hendrix, reaped the rewards of the sexual excitement with which they could inflame an audience. The same is true of some conductors, and at a more modest level of piano teachers. Dancing masters had a similar reputation in the eighteenth century; nor were Rudolf Nureyev and Salome without their admirers.

In his well-known line about the power of 'cheap music', Noel Coward exposes a truth in his usual self-mocking, insouciant manner. Songs, like perfumes, linger in the memory forever identified with a person or an event. Most songs are about love, and every love affair has its own song or its own piece of music.

Although 'music' means 'of the Muse' it was ultimately a gift to mankind from Apollo. In the beautiful myth of Orpheus and Eurydice, the sun god gives his lyre to Orpheus who plays so wonderfully that for a moment the birds stop singing, the winds cease blowing and the rivers no longer flow – so perfectly does Orpheus blend and harmonize the sounds of Nature. The maiden Eurydice is spellbound by the glorious music and she and Orpheus fall in love. But their happiness is short-lived. With echoes of another paradise lost, a serpent bites her and she dies, descending into the realms of death. Grief stricken, Orpheus follows her. His music so charms the grim gods of the underworld that they agree to release Eurydice. She can return with Orpheus to the world of the living if he promises not to look back at his lover until they are beyond the boundaries of Hades. In his happiness at being reunited with the only woman he has ever loved Orpheus forgets his promise and looks back. It is the last time he will ever see Eurydice.

The ancients believed that the haunting melodies created by Orpheus in his grief, were the origins of all the tunes with which lovers have since consoled themselves.

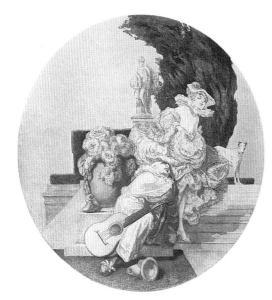

OPPOSITE PAGE: Greek dancer, origin
unknown
LEFT: Lithograph, Franz von Bayros

BELOW: *Orpheus and Eurydice*, Sir Edward
Poynter, 1836-1919

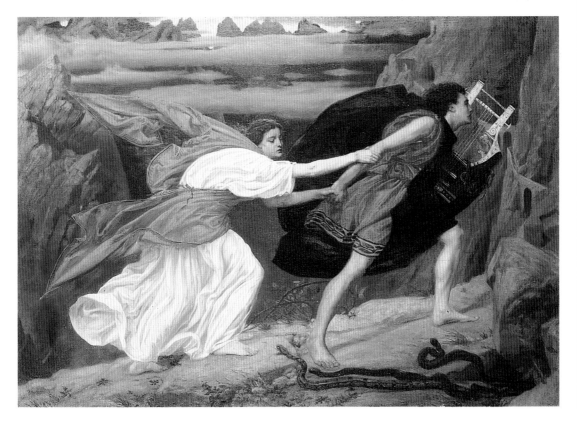

Although any piece of music can have erotic associations for a particular individual, and all music is sensually exciting in a way that could be described as sexual, some music is definitely erotic – and intended to be so. *Prélude à l'après-midi d'une faune* is an orchestral piece written by Claude Debussy (1862-1918) and based on a poem by the French symbolist poet Stéphane Mallarmé (1842-1898). Subtle and delicate, it follows the erotic

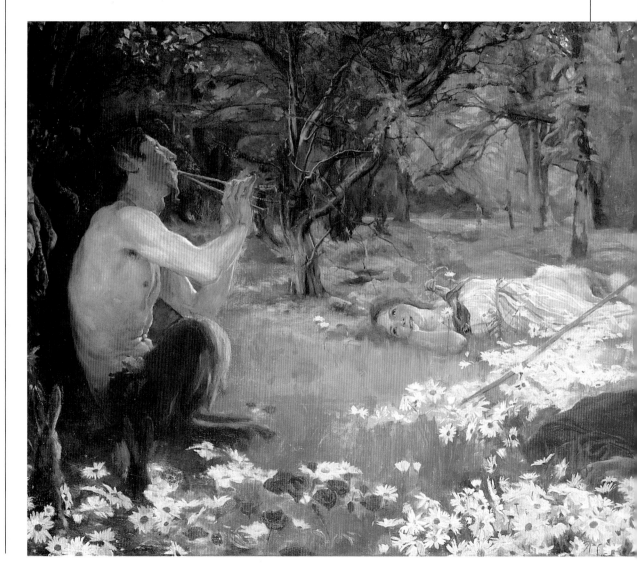

musings of a faun on a drowsy summer afternoon bathed in sunshine. The flute is used for the faun theme, and introduces the work; the theme is then taken up by oboe and clarinet. Fauns, or satyrs in Greek mythology, are the followers of the god Pan and it is appropriate that the orchestra has a rich woodwind section and horns, but no other brass or percussion (except cymbals).

LEFT: *Pan*, Gerald Fenwick Metcalfe, late nineteenth century

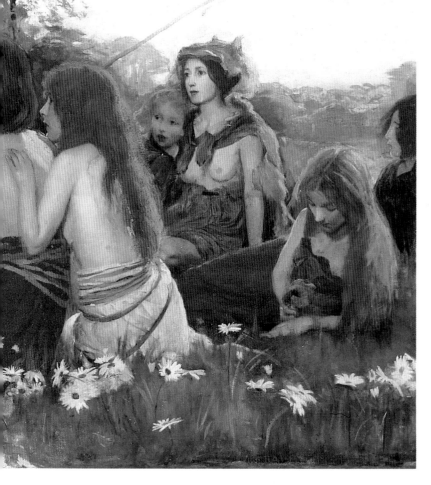

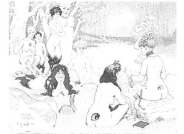

ABOVE: *Faune o'clock*, H. Gerbault, circa 1895

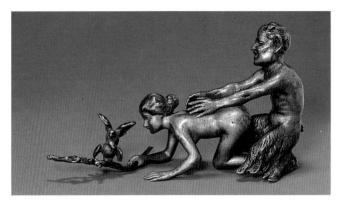

ABOVE: *Satyr with Nymph*, bronze, nineteenth century
BELOW: *The Wooing of Daphnis*, Arthur Lemon, 1850-1912
OPPOSITE PAGE, TOP AND BOTTOM: Engravings of Satyrs, eighteenth century

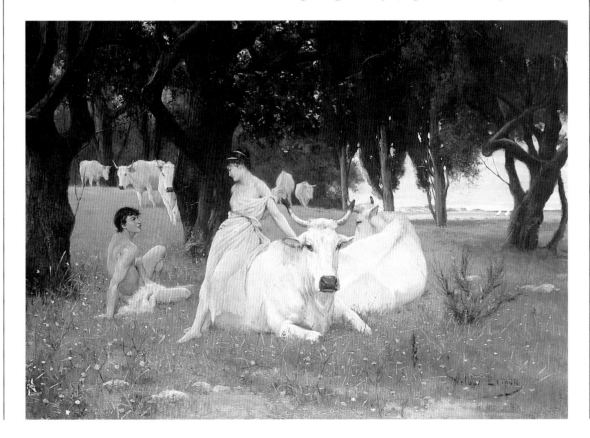

Bolero by Maurice Ravel (1875-1937) is often chosen as an example of erotic music. In this orchestral work the same theme is repeated throughout in one long crescendo. The first exposition of the theme is on flute, then clarinet, then bassoon accompanied by side drums, until the entire orchestra joins in, building to a tremendous orgasmic finish in which the earth definitely moves.

LE SATYRE
FAILLISSANT.

The ballet *Daphnis et Chloé* which Ravel wrote for Diaghilev's company in 1912 is no less sexy. Based on a tale by Longus written in the fourth century BC, it describes the tribulations of the shepherd Daphnis and his love, the shepherdess Chloé . When Chloé is kidnapped by pirates, Daphnis prays to the great god Pan for help. Assistance of another kind comes from the voracious Lykanion who seduces Daphnis in his lover's absence. But supernatural forces are at work: the statues of three nymphs come to life to give spiritual support, and when the pirate chief Bryaxis attempts to rape Chloé, the great god himself appears, chasing the villains who flee in literal 'panic'.

The famous sunrise music heralds the reunion of the lovers, who show their gratitude to Pan by re-enacting the story of Syrinx, a nymph the old goat once loved. A heady baccanale closes the work. All the music is earthy and powerfully sexual, not just the well-known concert suites but the entire work. Most erotic of all are the mystical nymph's dance, the seduction by Lykanion, and the whirling bacchanalia at the finish.

LE SATYRE ET SA FEMME .

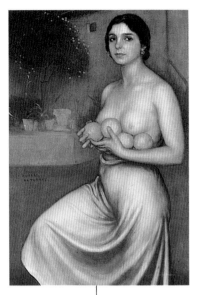

Andalucia, with its history, climate and unique mix of cultures, could make a reasonable claim to being the most sensuous place on earth. Manuel de Falla (1876-1946) conjures the erotic spirit of place in *Noches en los Jardines de Espana* (Nights in the Gardens of Spain), 'impressions' for piano and orchestra in three movements. The music is a magical evocation of hot, sultry nights: the air heavy with jasmine, animal scents and the odour of centuries. It takes you into dark patios, where the splash of cool water from unseen fountains is the sound made by the piano.

El Sombrero de Tres Picos (The Three-Cornered Hat) by the same composer is sexual in a more direct way. A miller and his beautiful wife outwit the lecherous Corregidor (magistrate); the miller's dance, a farucca, is a controlled explosion of concentrated machismo, slow but intense at first, then gaining speed rapidly like a lunging phallus. The famous Spanish dancer Antonio once made a virtuoso recording of the miller's dance complete with zapateado, the fierce foot stamping typical of gypsy flamenco.

Georges Bizet (1838-1875) was a Parisian, but he breathed life into the unforgettable Spanish gypsy Carmen. Based on the novel by Prosper Mérimée, the opera *Carmen* is set in Seville in the 1820s. Carmen (either mezzo or soprano) makes her first appearance singing the sinuous melody of the habanera: 'L'amour est un oiseau rebel'. The object of her sexual taunting is Don José, who affects indifference. But the swaying rhythm and Carmen's hips tell us otherwise: we know it cannot be long, as she circles him like a predatory cat. Death is the only possible release from the uncontrollable passions she releases, and it follows, as inevitable as Don José's seduction.

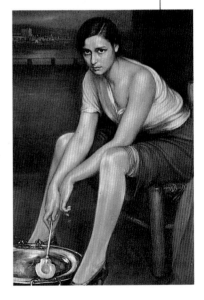

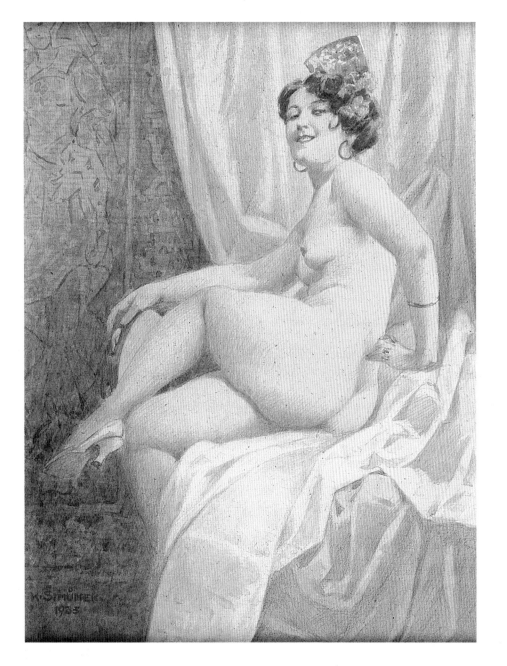

OPPOSITE PAGE: Naranjas y Limones, and Chiquita Piconera, Julio Romero de Torres, 1874-1930
ABOVE: *Gypsy*, K. Simunek, 1935

Like Carmen, the arch-seducer Don Juan is said to have lived in Seville. The story of this rapacious womanizer has been retold many times, but never better than by Wolfgang Amadeus Mozart (1756-1791) in his opera *Don Giovanni*, first performed in Prague in 1787. At the beginning of Act II, the great lover is joking with his servant Leporello who keeps the notorious list of the 1003 women Don Giovanni has enjoyed with details of their most intimate secrets. Catching sight of the maid of his former mistress Donna Elvira at her window, Don Giovanni sees an opportunity of adding a pretty young girl to his list. Whether he succeeds or not is never made clear, but it is difficult to imagine any woman resisting Mozart's seductive serenade. Taking a mandolin, Don Giovanni (baritone) sings:

Deh! vieni a la finestra, o mio tesoro;
Deh, vieni a consolar il pianto mio.
Se neghi a me di dar qualche ristoro,
Davanti agli occhi tuoi morir vogl'io.

Tu ch'hai la bocca dolce più del miele
Tu che il zucchero porti in mezzo al core
Non esser, gioia mia, con me crudele,
Lasciati almen veder, mio bell' amore!

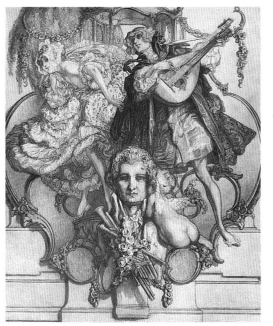

LEFT: Lithograph, Franz
von Bayros

BELOW: Nude, Paul François
Quinsac, born 1858
OPPOSITE PAGE: Drawing by
an unknown artist

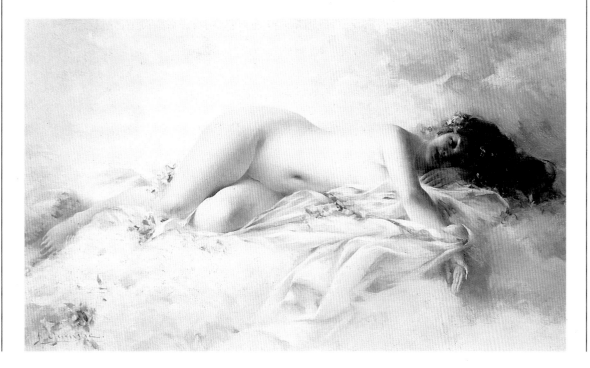

The two great German composers concerned with the themes of love and sex – and death – are Richard Wagner (1813-1883) and Richard Strauss (1864-1949). Wagner explored the dark side of eroticism in *Tristan and Isolde*, and his opera *Die Walküre* (The Valkyrie) also caused a sensation when it was first performed in Munich in 1870. The incestuous lovers, Siegmund and Sieglinde, are the earthling children of the god Wotan who have been separated since childhood. In Act I they meet and fall in love to a glorious, passionate duet ('bride and sister be to your brother'). In Act II Wotan's favourite daughter Brünnhilde – one of the nine warrior maidens or Valkyries born of

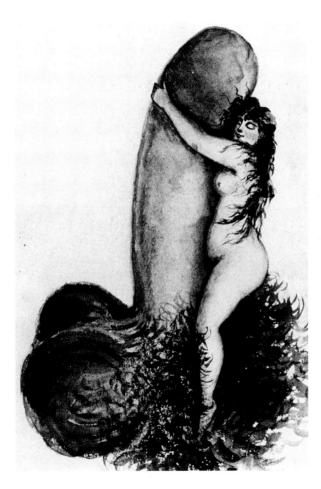

Wotan (sky) and Erda (earth) – is given her orders: she must allow Siegmund to die in battle. But when Brünnhilde tells Siegmund of his fate she is moved by his manly response and decides to help the unhappy pair by rescuing his wife Sieglinde who is now pregnant.

At the beginning of Act III comes the famous 'Ride of the Valkyries', when the other eight sisters await Brünnhilde who comes, not with the expected dead hero, but with Sieglinde on her saddle. All the Valkyries have flying horses to carry fallen warriors from the battlefield to Valhalla. Their 'Ride' – which is often played as a concert piece for orchestra

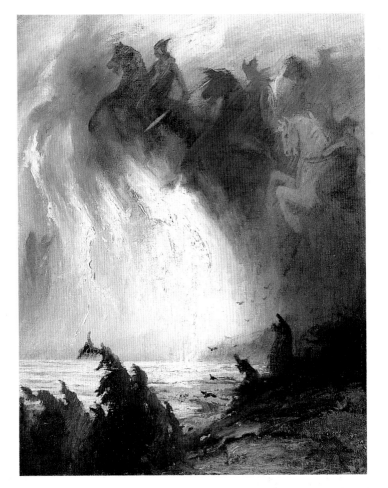

alone – is one of the most stirring pieces in all music, charged with animal lust and violent emotion: 'Go tether your chesnut/next to my grey/she will be glad/to graze by your stallion… your stallion is biting my mare!/see that the mares/are far from the stallions/until our heroes' hate is quenched!'

ABOVE: *The Ride of the Valkyries*, Hermann Hendrich, born 1856
OPPOSITE PAGE: Drawing by an unknown artist, nineteenth century

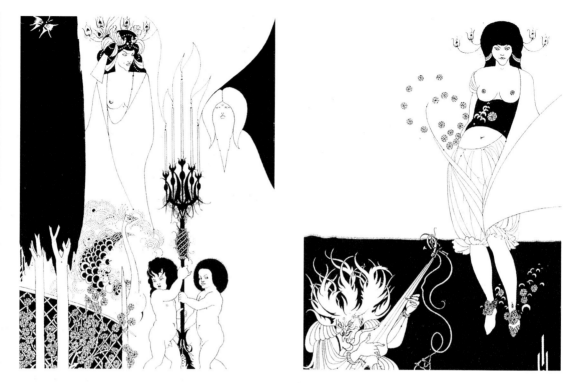

Salome – the one-act opera first performed in Dresden in 1905 – is Richard Strauss's exploration of the dark shadows of eroticism. The libretto is based on Oscar Wilde's play, and deals with the familiar story of King Herod, so obsessed with his stepdaughter that he grants her any wish if she will dance for him. Salome, who did have a less than ideal home environment, then performs the most famous striptease in history, but demands the head of John the Baptist as her reward. Strauss's music is richly sensuous and suitably decadent. 'The Dance of the Seven Veils' has an oriental flavour, with a sinuous thread of melody on the oboe and other woodwind weaving its way through the orchestra.

In *Der Rosenkavalier* (The Knight of the Rose), written five years after Salome, Strauss comes out of the shadows and into the sunlight. *Der Rosenkavalier* is the bitter-sweet story of an older woman and her young lover, whom she generously releases when he finds a more appropriate love. It is a warm, humane work, which celebrates sexuality. The short orchestral introduction is an explicit description of the lovemaking of the Marschallin (soprano) and Count Octavian (a mezzo-soprano travesti role) which continues as the curtain rises. The music is passionate and excited, with an outburst from the horns at the critical moment, dissolving into a post-coital glow.

In quite different mood is the trio for female voices at the end of *Der Rosenkavalier.* This thrilling climax epitomizes Strauss's 'love affair with the female voice' and sets the hair and everything else on end.

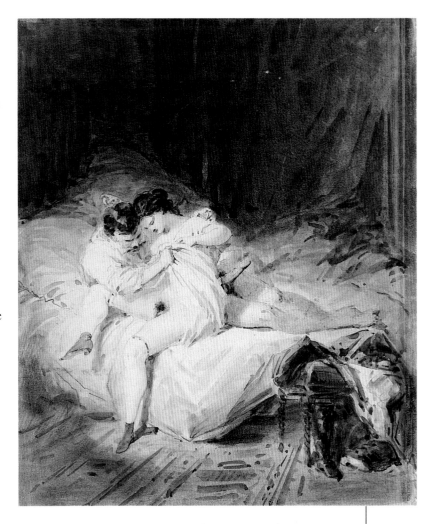

OPPOSITE PAGE, LEFT: *The Eyes of Herod*, Aubrey Beardsley
OPPOSITE PAGE, RIGHT: *The Stomach Dance*, Aubrey Beardsley
ABOVE: Watercolour, Edouard de Beaumont, 1821-1888

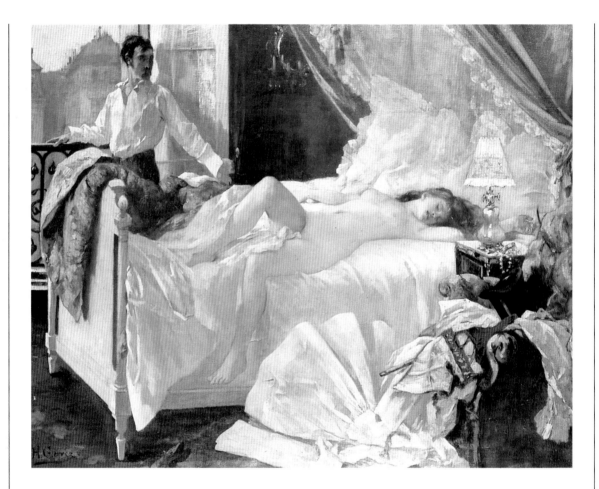

ABOVE: *Rolla*, Henri Gervex, 1852-1929
OPOSITE PAGE: *Lithograph*, Nicolas F.O.Tassaert, 1800-1874

Also Sprach Zarathustra (1896) by Richard Strauss is probably the most uncompromisingly phallic work in music; but for a more satisfying and complicated 'maleness' there is nothing better than the third movement of the 'Waldstein' (piano sonata no. 21 in C , opus 53) by Ludwig van Beethoven (1770-1827). It is a technically brilliant and demanding piece: joyous and positive, fierce and thrusting, moving swiftly from loud to soft, then back again. There is a resolution towards the end, when the pianist

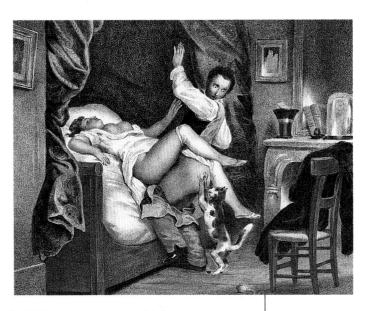

climbs effortfully up the scale and comes out into the light – a moment which a woman writer describes as 'turning the insides to water'.

Our response to music is as personal and individual as our response to sex. If your erotic music is epitomized by the trumpet of Miles Davis, or the rubato style of Frank Sinatra, or the Italian bel canto tradition, or any of the thousand rock children of Rhythm and Blues – you might still find a few sexual surprises among the following:

Fréderick Chopin: *Grand Polonaise*

Richard Wagner: *Tristan und Isolde*, Liebestod (love duet in Act II)

Maurice Ravel: *L'enfant et les Sortilèges* (cat duet at end of Scene I)

Carl Orff: *Carmina Burana* (especially the beginning)

Camille Saint-Saëns: *Samson et Dalila*, baccanale

Heitor Villa-Lobos: *Bachianas Brasileiras*

Igor Stravinsky: *The Rite of Spring* (especially the Sacrificial Dance at the end)

Béla Bartók: *Duke Bluebeard's Castle*

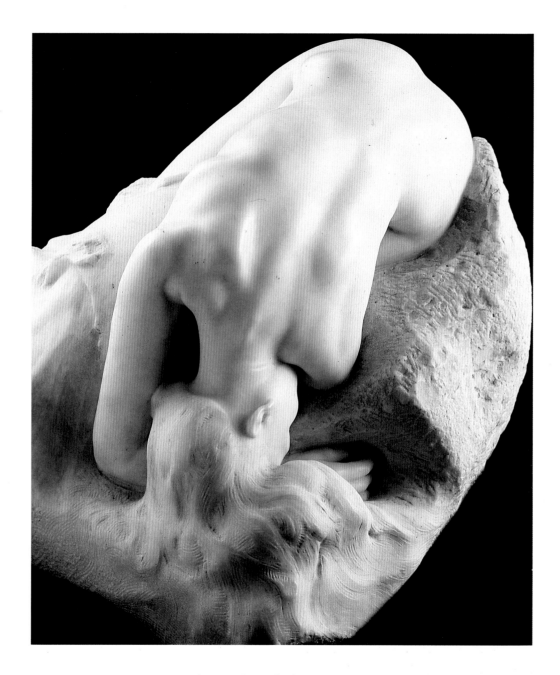

ABOVE: *Danaide*, August Rodin
OPPOSITE: Mother of pearl carving, Netherlands, late seventeenth century

T O U C H

(O)nly touch can make the world completely real: it is the first and last link which connects us to life and to each other. 'Keep in touch' we say; 'Let us not lose touch'. And if our emotions are affected by something, we say that it is 'touching'. It is the most basic of all the senses, the foundation: it is also the most generous and compassionate.

'...she was crying blindly, in all the anguish of her generation's forlornness. His heart melted suddenly, like a drop of fire, and he put out his hand and laid his fingers on her knee.

'You shouldn't cry,' he said softly.

But then she put her hands over her face and felt that really her heart was broken and nothing mattered any more. He laid his hand on her shoulder, and softly, gently, it began to travel down the curve of her back, blindly, with a blind stroking motion, to the curve of her crouching loins. And there his hand softly, softly, stroked the curve of her flank, in the blind instinctive caress.'

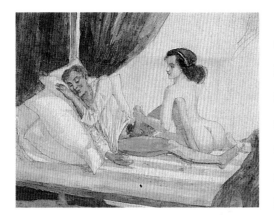

'She lay quite still, in a sort of sleep, in a sort of dream. Then she quivered as she felt his hand groping softly, yet with queer thwarted clumsiness, among her clothing. Yet the hand knew, too, how to unclothe her where it wanted. He drew down the thin silk sheath, slowly, carefully, right down and over her feet. Then with a quiver of exquisite pleasure he touched the warm soft body...'

Lady Chatterley's Lover

Hands are our most loyal servants, we expect them to do anything and everything – and they do. Civilization was conceived by the human brain, but it was human hands which made it a reality. So it is with sex, where our hands go before us not so much as erotic diplomats more as viceroys:

Licence my roving hands, and let them go
Before, behind, between, above, below.
Oh, my America, my new-found-land,
My kingdom, safest when with one man mann'd,
My mine of precious stones, my empery;
How am I blest in thus discovering thee!
To enter in these bonds, is to be free;
Then, where my hand is set, my seal shall be.

From *Going to Bed*, John Donne

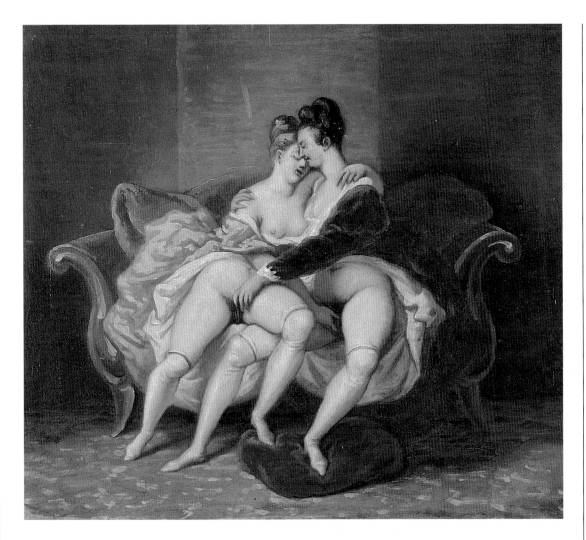

OPPOSITE PAGE: Watercolour by 'Fay D' circa 1920

ABOVE: *Tender Girlfriend*s, attributed to Michael Martin Drolling, 1786-1851

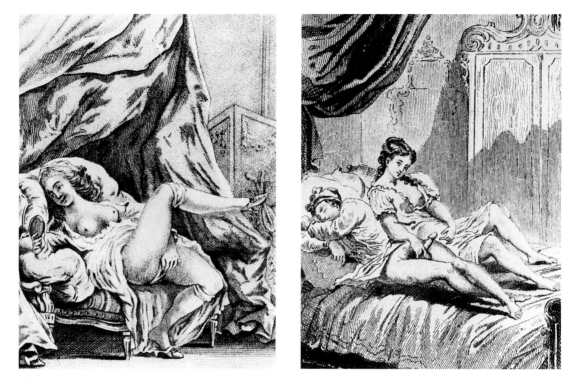

The first erotic journeys our hands make are, of course, to explore ourselves. It is a pleasant journey for all its limitations, which is just as well because on joining the human race we are each given a life-long season ticket. There is an old joke that '95 per cent of males and 85 per cent of females masturbate; and that five per cent of males and fifteen per cent of females lie about it'. Why should anyone lie about an activity as normal as eating? Although if you do it with the same frequency as eating it probably is best to lie about it. Masturbation is the very necessary journey of self-exploration we make before going on to more satisfying and demanding journeys with other people. We will make solitary excursions again, throughout life, if we are lonely or even if we are not. The latter does not imply lack of satisfaction with a partner, it is simply a different aspect of our sexuality. Lovers who do not understand this and feel inadequate or rejected should learn to masturbate their partner as well as he or she does (although most women would agree

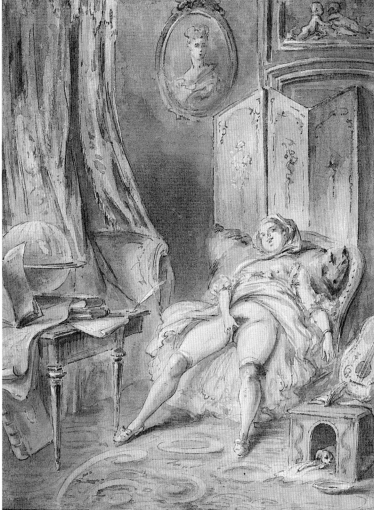

that the tongue is mightier than the finger in this respect). Throughout history all the great courtesans, however grand, have known the value of manual labour.

ABOVE: *Lonely pleasures,* After Pierre-Antoine Baudouin, 1723-1769
OPPOSITE PAGE, LEFT AND RIGHT: French engravings, eighteenth century

Masturbation is a gift which all lovers exchange, sometimes simultaneously, as part of their lovemaking or instead of it. It can become the most intimate form of theatre yet devised, or it can be solitary. Images of women masturbating are probably the most frequently reproduced icons in erotic art, which shows the power of the idea in the male imagination. Yet despite all this, masturbation in its solitary form carries with it an absurd legacy of guilt. The word itself derives from the Latin manu stuprare, meaning 'to defile oneself with the hand'. The Roman writers Juvenal and Martial condemned the practice, while the Greeks went to the other extreme, with the philosopher Chrysippus praising Diogenes for doing it in the market-place! Scholars continued to debate (and, no doubt, to masturbate) throughout the Christian period. Theodore of Tarsus (602-690) thought 'forty days penance' appropriate while Caramuel declared more sensibly 'natural law does not forbid masturbation'.

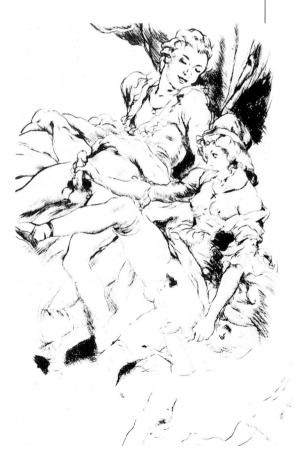

The Victorians made an extraordinary fuss about what they called 'self abuse'. Britain's sporting heritage can be regarded as a vast conspiracy to divert the energies of young people

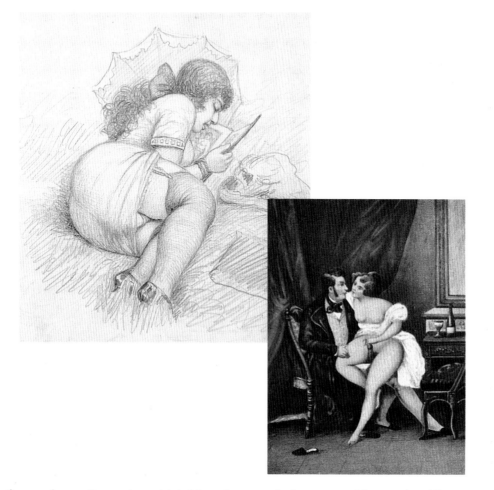

away from a form of exercise which Victorian quack doctors – with no scientific

justification – blamed for blindness, insanity and a host of other disorders.

ABOVE RIGHT: Coloured engraving, artist unknown, nineteenth century
ABOVE LEFT: Pencil drawing, Italy, circa 1930
OPPOSITE PAGE, TOP: Drawing by Leporini, contemporary
OPPOSITE PAGE, BOTTOM: Illustration by 'Schem', France, circa 1920

The early twentieth-century reaction to disabling Victorian ideas about sex, such as the lies and nonsense written about masturbation, is not without its lighter side. In the chapter on 'auto-erotism' in his *Psychology of Sex,* Havelock Ellis while demonstrating the guiltlessness and normality of masturbation, also achieves moments of high comedy. We are told how elephants masturbate (with their trunks, naturally) and how female ferrets do (with small round stones). The entire animal kingdom, both male and female – from Welsh ponies to peewits, and parrots to camels – turns out to be full of ingenious and inveterate masturbators. We feel rather sorry for the lonely bear who played with himself when he saw other bears coupling, and wonder at the lascivious ingenuity of goats who fellate themselves.

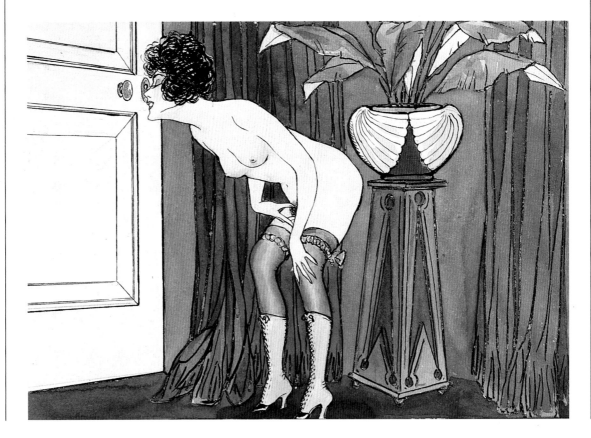

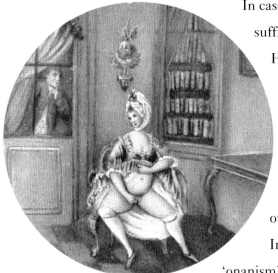

In case parallels in animal behaviour are not sufficient to rid masturbation of its bad name, Havelock Ellis also lists the great and the good of our own species who have either admitted to it or been observed enjoying it. The male list includes Rousseau, Goethe, Gogol and Kierkegaard, while anonymous female worthies describe their own intimate behaviour in luxurious detail.

In many European languages variants of 'onanism' are the preferred word for auto-sexual practices. This term takes its name from the biblical character Onan (*Genesis* 38:9) who may have preferred to make his mark on history in some different way. The writer and wit Dorothy Parker (1893-1967) had a caged bird she called Onan. When asked why, she replied 'because he spills his seed on the ground'.

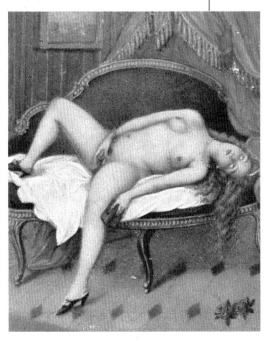

ABOVE AND RIGHT: Illustrations from a nineteenth century erotic novel
OPPOSITE PAGE: Coloured drawing, artist unknown.

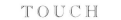

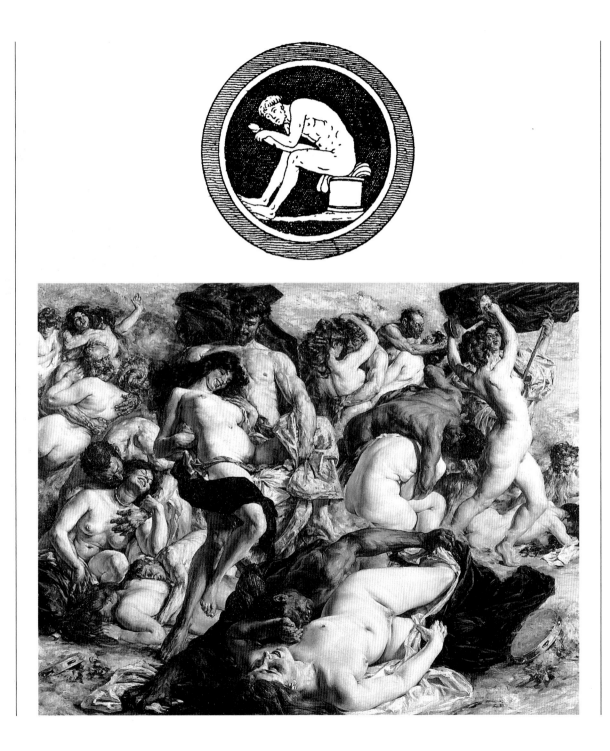

The ringing biblical phrase 'the sins of the flesh' is often used to describe sensual (and in particular sexual) pleasure by those opposed to it for religious, moral or envious reasons. The elusive and surreal 'flesh pots' are closely related. Whatever we may think about the metaphors and proscriptions of Old Testament prophets, they were absolutely right about the flesh.

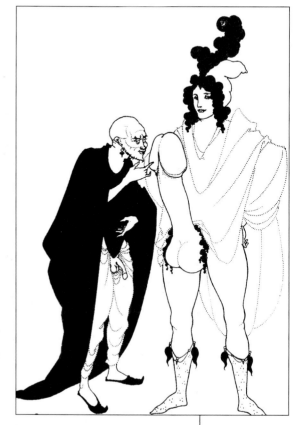

Our skin is the largest organ in the body, which it both defines and protects. Because the skin is generously provided with sense receptors – more than 9,000 per square inch on the exquisitely sensitive fingertips – we can both give and receive pleasure, by touching and being touched. The hairless, and often more darkly pigmented structures – penis tip, lips, tongue, nipples, clitoris etc. – are particularly well-served with high concentrations of the most sensitive cells, which is why we derive so much pleasure from bringing them all into contact with one another.

The so-called 'erogenous zones' of the body can be a limiting idea. Some men if asked to draw a diagrammatic male body with the size of organs corresponding to their erogenous significance would produce something similar in proportion – if not in artistic execution – to Aubrey Beardsley's *Herald Examined*. Popular parlance provides an appropriate and pithy description of the penis-oriented male...

ABOVE: *The Herald Examined,* from Lysistrata, Aubrey Beardsley
OPPOSITE PAGE, BOTTOM: *A Bacchanalian Scene,* August Leveque, 1864-1921
OPPOSITE PAGE, TOP: *Priapus,* neo-classical, origin unknown

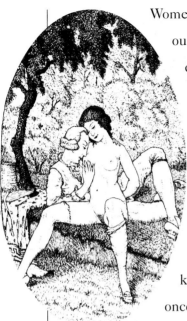

Women are more likely than men to appreciate the importance of widening our skin eroticism to include the whole body: the clitoris being less credible than a penis as a peg on which to hang all one's hopes for sexual fulfilment. Although we do sometimes learn bad habits from our sexual partners in our eagerness to please, and for every bully-boy penis there is a clitoris who is a martinet.

The entire body surface, in men and in women, has erotic potential. We learn the obvious places in childhood with tickling and then tend to forget that we can revisit the same sites with quite different intentions as adults. The soles of the feet, the backs of knees, below the arms and the neck, all yearn for kisses and caresses, as once they dreaded tickles.

Toes that once wriggled pleasurably in sand or mud can be nibbled (it is even called 'shrimping') as can earlobes. More directly erotic are the insides of the thighs and the perineum which are extremely sensitive to touch, and breasts and buttocks whose sense receptors respond to kneading: gentle for the former, vigorous for the latter.

'Give her your jasmine for the dance girls, then lie her gently back and, pressing a paan between her lips and making sure her cup is kept well-filled, massage her body with sweet sandal oil. Soon she won't object to fingers that stray under her skirt-hem and linger at her lightly-knotted waistband; when her eyes are dreamy and her breathing's harsh, send the servants away.'

Kama Sutra, Mallyana Vatsyayana

ABOVE: Engraving, M.E.Phillipp
OPPOSITE PAGE: Bronze figure of the goddess Parvati, India, seventeenth century

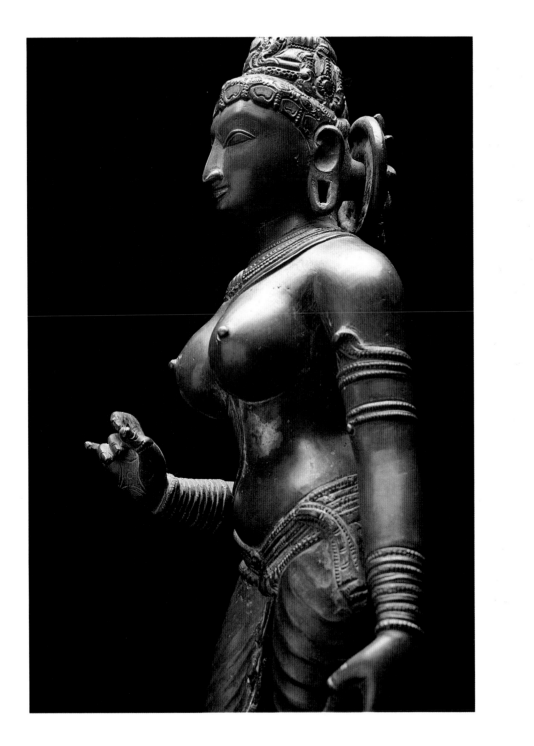

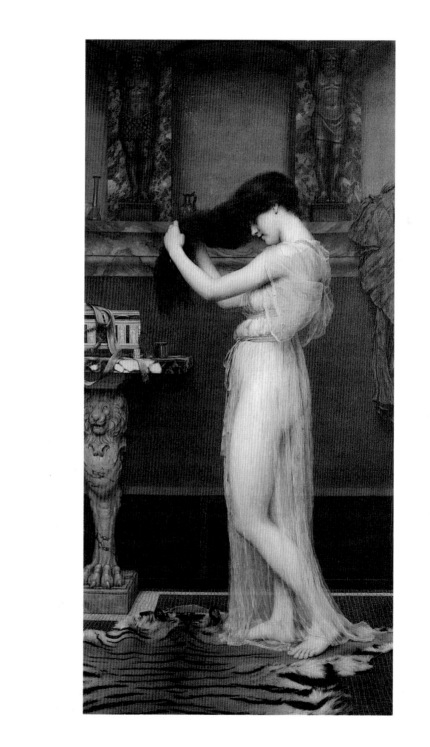

Hair, as we have already seen, provides us with our own scented powder puffs (underarms and pubis) and incense burner (head) as well as dramatizing the appearance of our bodies. It has one more erotic trick. Every hair – and our bodies are covered with millions of them ranging from nearly invisible fine down to structures like pine trees in comparison – is also wired in to our nervous system. Because of hair, large areas of our bodies are intensely sensitive: the lightest touch of a lover's fingertip sends a forest fire of sensation sweeping across our flesh. Head hair too, can be the source of great pleasure – both for the stroker and the stroked.

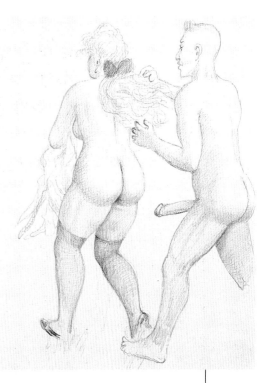

The very real sexual significance of hair is probably the origin of the mystical associations it gathered as it wound its way through different cultures. In the strange tale of Samson and Delilah (*Judges* 16) there is sufficient mention of harlots and other women before Delilah to suggest that the vigour which the Israelite hero lost because of an unsympathetic haircut was not restricted to the battlefield. Medieval witches had their heads shaved in the belief that it removed their power: in fact they were being unsexed. Similar thoughts were probably in St Paul's mind when he said 'if a man have long hair, it is a shame unto him' (I *Corinthians* II.14); although he was himself naturally bald, which can indicate high levels of the male sex hormone testosterone.

Opposite Page: *The Toilet,* John William Godward, 1861-1922
Above: Pencil drawing by an unknown Italian artist, circa 1920

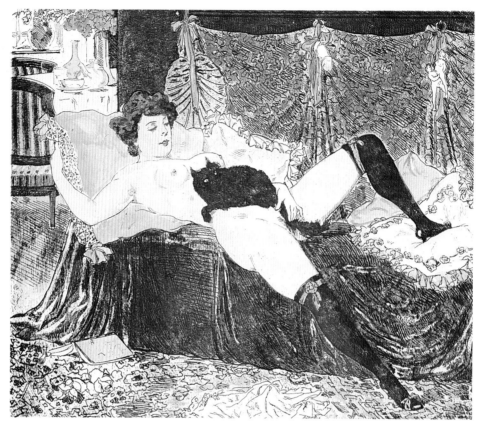

Our sense of touch is such a powerful channel for erotic stimuli that we borrow tactile experiences from other species and invent new, artificial ones. Our borrowings include fur – which is as beautiful to look at as it is to touch – and feathers, which we use mainly for display, but which also have tactile applications. Ironically, both fur and feathers are also part of the tactile equipment of the animals from which they come. With the advent of synthetic fur we no longer need to feel guilty about the fate of the donor which is likely to be a North Sea oil rig.

Leather can also be replicated artificially but, as with fur, our own sensitive skin (and our sense of sight and smell) can always tell the difference. Many people find wearing leather comfortable and pleasurable – and sexually exciting to a greater or lesser degree.

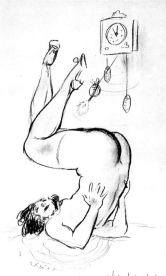

Rubber is best left to sub-aqua enthusiasts and dedicated fetishists, but PVC has a mainstream following although it is on the borderline. Perhaps its borderline position is the key to the appeal which PVC clothing has for some people, exploring the grey (or black and shiny) area between the tarty and the chic, the fetishistic and the acceptable.

OPPOSITE PAGE: Book illustration, early twentieth century
LEFT: Erotic postcard, circa 1930
BOTTOM: *Bearskin rug,* Raphaël Kirchner

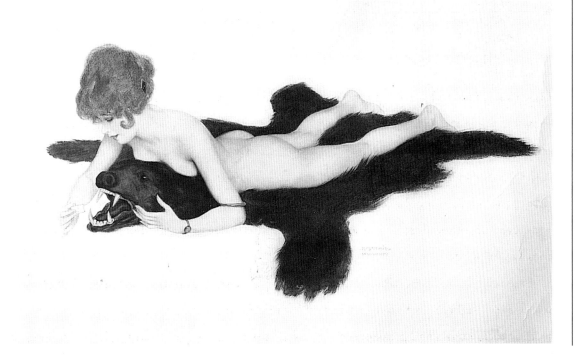

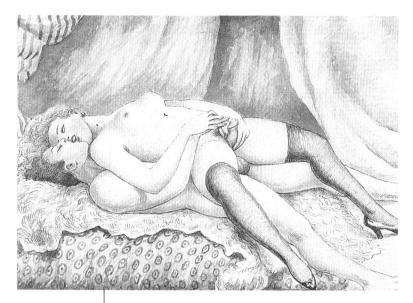

As with all the other senses, our erotic imagination has devised additional ways of enjoying the sense of touch. Lovemaking à L'Espagnol, or intra mammary intercourse, stimulates a woman's breasts and nipples, while offering an alternative venue for the adventurous penis. Armpits can be used in the same way with suitable lubrication, as can buttocks or the sensitive flesh between the thighs. Naturally enough, lovemaking between buttocks and thighs tends to lead to penetration. Zulu warriors and maidens were traditionally permitted to enjoy one another by moving the penis between the girls' thighs (intra femora) which they called 'the wiping of the spears'. The intention of the Zulu elders was to prevent unwanted pregnancies – an aim in which they were often unsuccessful since the greatest of all their warrior kings, the mighty Chaka, was conceived in this way.

Skin eroticism of a less obvious kind is the secret agenda of the innocent pendant earring, which stimulates the erogenous earlobe by constantly tugging at it while at the same time exciting the sensitive skin surface of the neck. Many of our body adornments combine display with tactile stimulation.

TOP: Watercolour by an unknown artist, circa 1930
BOTTOM: Charcoal drawing by 'A1', Vienna, 1933
OPPOSITE PAGE: *A Beauty*, Eugene de Blaas, 1843-1931

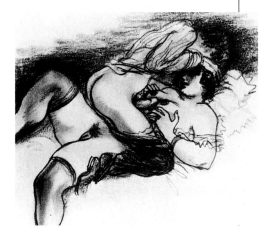

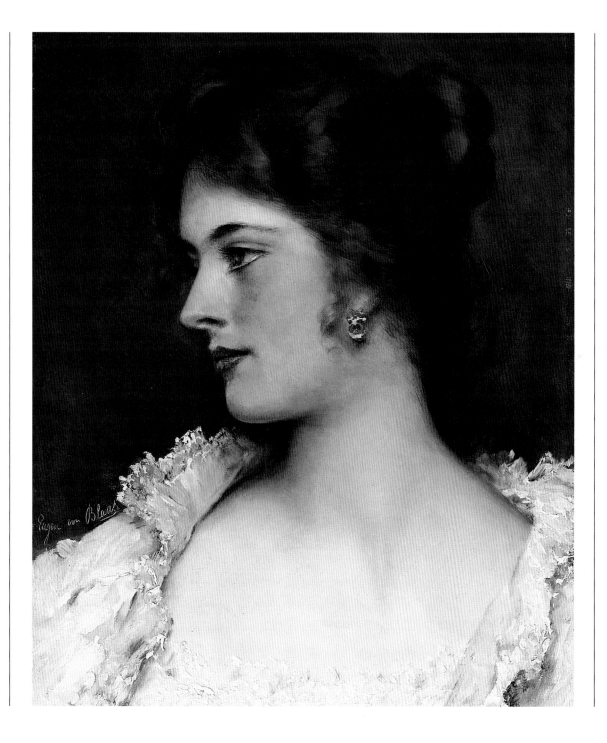

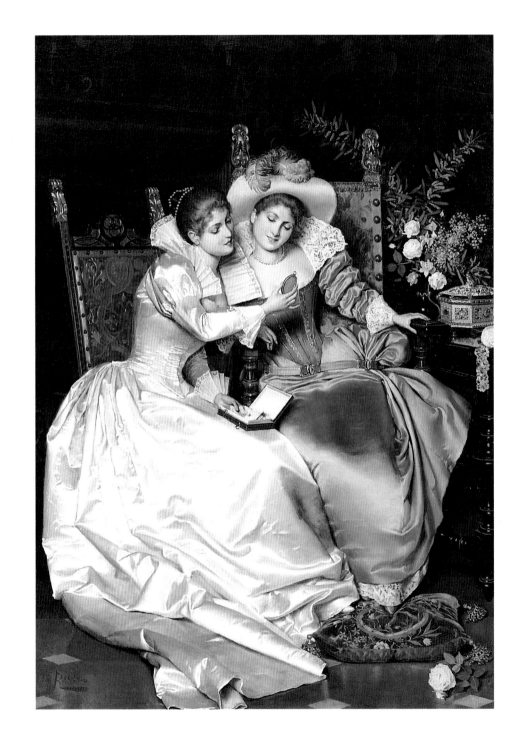

Textiles with which we come into contact must of course please our eyes with their colour and pattern, but they must also give us tactile pleasure. Contemporary clothing offers few of the luxurious combinations of surface and texture, and visual extravagance, which were once available in the clothes of wealthy men and women. But what our senses of touch and sight have lost, we have gained olfactorily with the benefits of dry cleaning and washable fabrics.

The most sensual textiles – silks, satins, velvet and cashmere – are also the most refined and therefore the most expensive. They are pleasing to touch because they imitate – and make us recall subliminally – the surfaces of our own bodies. Silk is like the finest human hair or the skin of a breast. Velvet is a downy bottom or a soft cheek; satin, the shiny glans of an engorged penis miraculously made available by the yard.

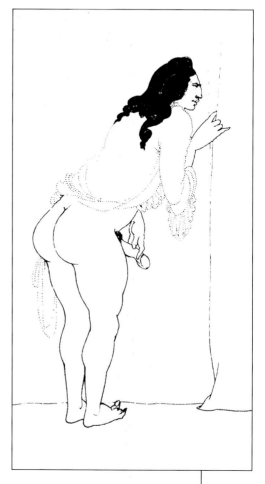

Cotton and synthetic substitutes have gone a long way to replacing linen on our tables and our beds. Naturally, there has been a corresponding fall in the number of linen fetishists who were once legion. But as any one of the few who remain would no doubt confirm, nothing can compare with a fine old linen sheet as a surface on which to make love.

OPPOSITE PAGE: *Admiring the Locket*, Pio Ricci, 1850-1919
TOP: *The Impatient Adulterer,* from Les Liaisons Dangereuses, Aubrey Beardsley

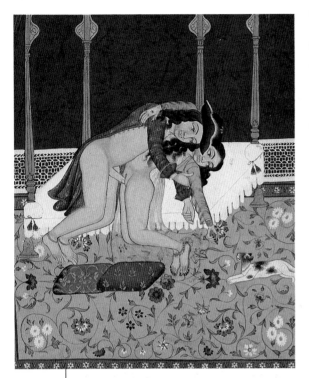

The bed is the most important piece of furniture in any house, yet often it is the most neglected. Each bed has its own individual character: it suggests different modes of lovemaking and makes its contribution to the sensations we feel. One of the many joys of travel is sampling the erotic possibilities of different beds, and the infinite range of tactile experiences they offer. Old hotels are preferable in many ways. Among the most important advantages they have over modern establishments, where everything is standardized, is the variety of beds provided. While touring you can make love on an engulfing marshmallow one night, and find yourselves on a trampoline the next.

Footboards and headboards offer different possibilities for the athletically inclined; brass beds are for animal impressions; four-posters for high drama – or farce.

The height of beds is important too. An old bed, like an old madam, will soon whisper the particular delights she has to offer: 'Kneel on the floor and you will be just the right height for prolonged, comfortable cunnilingus'; 'If you kneel on the bed he will be able to take you from behind while standing'.

ABOVE: *A Westerner with a Courtesan,* India, eighteenth century
OPPOSITE PAGE, BOTTOM: *Sweet Dreams,* Charles Chaplin, 1825-1891
OPPOSITE PAGE, TOP: Chinese watercolour, early nineteenth century

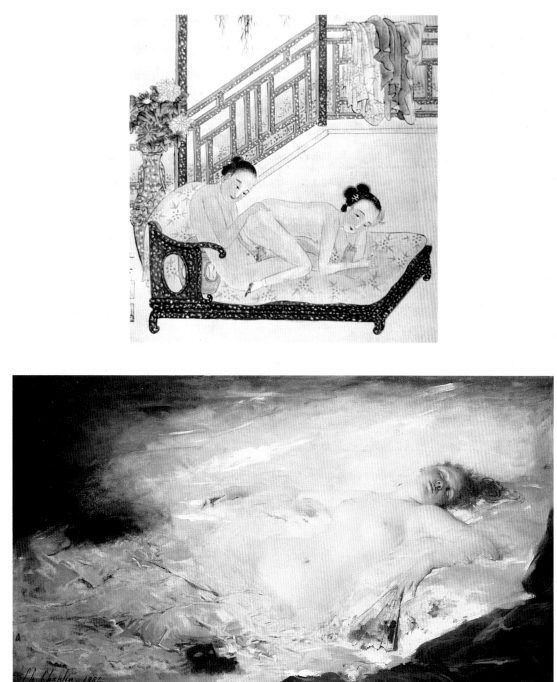

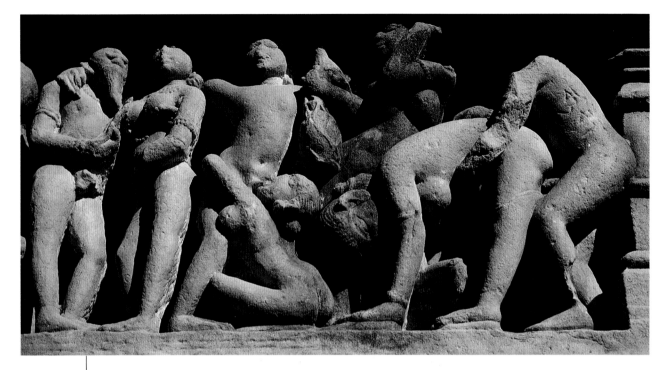

Sexual postures – and the fascination they hold for many people – have been a great blessing for stonemasons and woodcarvers, artists and engravers, writers, printers and publishers, down the ages. The most basic positions occur naturally and spontaneously to even the most uncreative lovers, and at first it is hard to see how a minor industry was created. As in so many things, we must look to the East for enlightenment, and in particular to India.

The Arab erotologist Sheikh Nefzawi readily admitted 'it is incontestable that the Hindus have surmounted enormous difficulties in coition'. But he goes on to say of a particular Indian posture: 'I think it is only realizable in thought or design'. The wily old Sheikh is right of course. The more preposterous positions illustrated by Indian miniaturists, which have been copied and re-copied in the bazaars for centuries and clearly found their way from Mughal India to Tunisia, were meant to amuse and titillate, nothing more. There are images of gymnastic sexual contortions which represent real asanas which only yogic or tantric adepts could, or would want, to achieve but these are in the minority.

The list of Hindu sexual postures which remains after we have eliminated the ludicrous and the mystical is still vast. One reason for this is that having no real analytical science, the ancient Hindus created lists. Lists tend to be sub-divided, and each new commentator will inevitably add refinements of his own while renaming old favourites. When this process is carried out over two millenia in a culture that takes sexual scholarship seriously, it is not surprising that the bemused inheritors of this accumulated wisdom assume there to be as many ways of making love as there are stars in the firmament. The real Indian contribution is not to be measured in volume: it is that they took sex seriously, realizing that it is at the very heart of everything. Furthermore, they embodied that religious belief in the importance of sex in sublime, guiltless art.

OPPOSITE PAGE: Stone frieze, Khajuraho temple, tenth century
BOTTOM: Mixed media painting, Bombay, contemporary

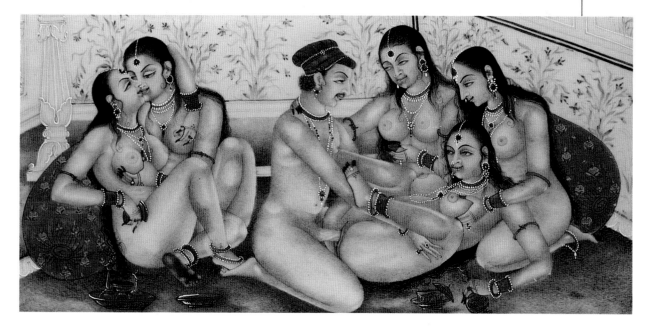

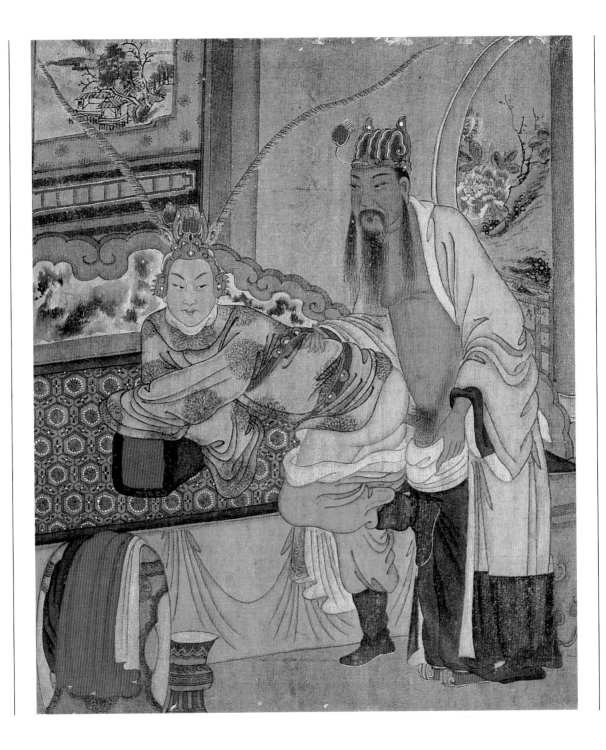

China's comprehensive sex manuals, which were produced over a long period, placed less emphasis on postures than the Hindu tradition but gave them delightful names such as 'Crossing the Mountains with Fire' (rear entry with external ejaculation) and 'Wailing Monkey Climbing a Tree' (man standing, woman's arms encircling his neck and legs around his waist). Fellatio was known as 'Playing the Jade Flute'. In both China and Japan, perhaps because high levels of personal hygiene were achieved at an early date, various anal practices were (and are) popular.

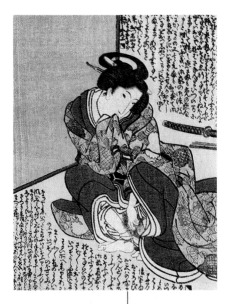

In Japan great emphasis has always been placed on sex toys, and many of the early manuals illustrate a bewildering array of gadgets and devices which men and women could use on themselves or to please each other. All too often, lonely courtesans and geishas, in a male-dominated society where lovers and clients were often absent, had to find what solace they could in rin-no-tama. These masturbation balls generated little shock waves as they knocked together in the user, who rocked in a chair or swing.

> The device of the two copper plums
>
> With silver in them
>
> Slowly and very slowly
>
> Satisfies. Just as all finishes
>
> Dew falls on my drenched hand.
>
> I would rather the bean flowered yellow
>
> And he were here!

Seventeenth-century Geisha poem

OPPOSITE PAGE: Painting on silk, China, circa 1700
TOP: Illustration from a Japanese Pillow Book

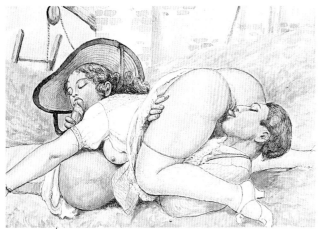

The publication of Sir Richard Burton's translation of *Kama Sutra* in 1883 rekindled a serious interest in sexual postures and other refinements of pleasure in the West. It was this new attitude which led, finally, to Alex Comfort's 1972 classic *The Joy of Sex* and all the imitations – some good, some not – which that has spawned.

Before *Kama Sutra*, the West's ideas about increasing sexual interest and enjoyment by using different positions were either spontaneous; or word-of-mouth recommendations; or postures gleened from the engraved illustrations to erotica. These illustrations included endless reconstructions of Aretino's 'Postures' of 1527, the original sixteen plates for which the *Sonnetti Lussuriosi* were written having been lost.

Prior to the Renaissance, a void stretches back across fourteen centuries to Ovid, whose *Art of Love* was written in the first century:

> …venerum jungunt per mille figuras,
> inveniat plures nulla tabella modus…

> 'They unite in Love in a thousand postures;
> no picture could suggest any new ones.'

Ovid is referring to the shadowy figure of the Greek woman Elephantis whose legendary writings on sexual positions inspired the erotic murals in the bedroom of the Emperor Tiberius.

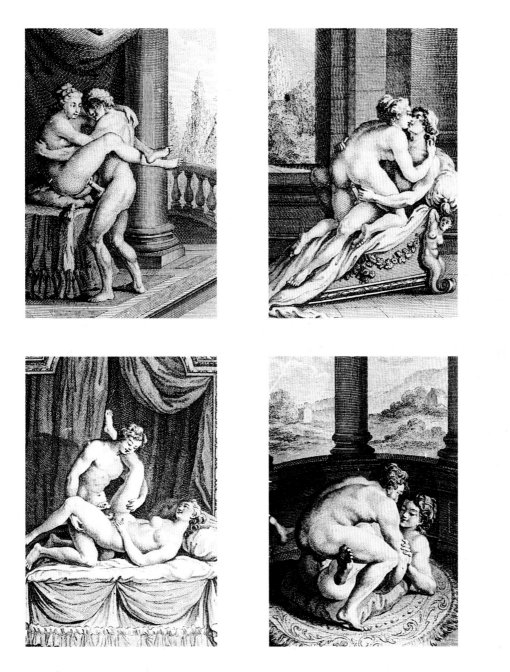

ABOVE: Engravings of sexual postures, eighteenth century
OPPOSITE PAGE: Watercolour by an unknown artist, circa 1930

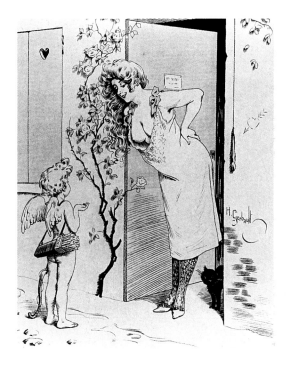

ABOVE: Drawing by H.Gerbault

BELOW: *Venus and Cupid,* Luis Riccardo Falero, 1851-1896

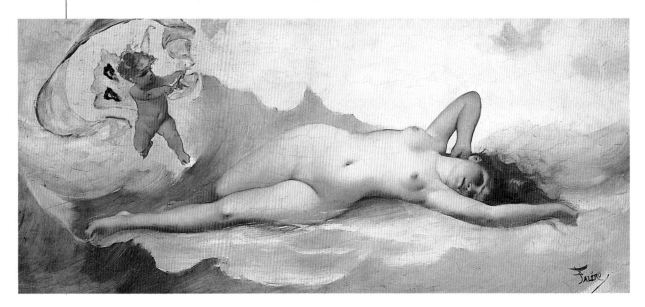

The Cloacae – Rome's great sewers – were presided over by Cloacina, an aspect of the love goddess Venus. The close identification of the two goddesses can be regarded either as a bad joke or as a useful reminder of the dual function of our sex organs and their close proximity to those concerned with waste disposal.

It is not difficult to see why human beings developed strong taboos around the inevitable consequences of eating and drinking, but that should not by association make us disgusted with any part of our bodies. Providing we are scrupulous in making regular devotions to the goddess Hygeia as well, no part of our body is disagreeable – or out of bounds in bed. Lady Chatterley's philosopher gamekeeper Mellors had the right idea:

> 'He stroked her tail with his hand, long and subtly taking in the curves and the globe-fullness.
>
> 'Tha's got such a nice tail on thee,' he said, in the throaty caressive dialect. 'Tha's got the nicest arse of anybody. It's the nicest, nicest woman's arse as is! An ivery bit of it is woman... Tha's got a real soft sloping bottom on thee, as a man loves in 'is guts. It's a bottom as could hold the world up, it is!'
>
> All the while he spoke he exquisitely stroked the rounded tail, till it seemed as if a slippery sort of fire came from it into his hands. And his finger-tips touched the two secret openings to her body, time after time, with a soft little brush of fire.
>
> 'An' if tha shits an' if tha pisses, I'm glad. I don't want a woman as couldna shit nor piss.'

Mellors is quite right, although the endearment of telling a lover she has 'a bottom as could hold the world up' is not likely to catch on. We are back to the Cloacae, which Pliny said made Rome 'suspended between heaven and earth'. If the gods have played a joke on us, it is very important that we have the last laugh.

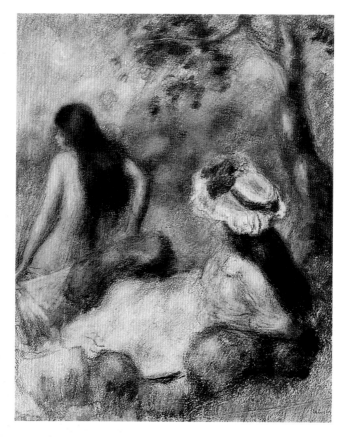

Water runs through every aspect of human life. The great rivers gave birth to our civilization, which still needs it just as every living thing does. We drink it, and we wash our bodies which are largely composed of water, in it. You might think we had had enough of water. But no, at every chance we swim and play in and on the water. What is the reason for this abiding passion? Is Sandor Ferenczi's Freudian theory correct, that within each of us there lies a deep-seated urge to return to the primeval ocean, from which an ancestor we would not immediately recognize crawled aeons ago?

There is an alternative explanation. Water is sexy. In this extract from the *Memoirs of a Woman of Pleasure*, Fanny Hill gives her own testimony:

'… the no more than grateful coolness of the water gave my senses a delicious refreshment from the sultriness of the season, and made me more alive, more happy in myself, and, in course, more alert, and open to voluptuous impressions… and now, nothing would serve him but giving his hands the regale of going over every part of me, neck, breast, belly, thighs and all the rest, so dear to the imagination, under the pretext of washing and rubbing them; as we both stood in the water, no higher now than the pit of our stomachs, and which did not hinder him from feeling, and toying with that leak that distinguishes our sex. And it is wonderfully water-light: for his fingers, in vain dilating and opening it, only let more flame than water into it…'

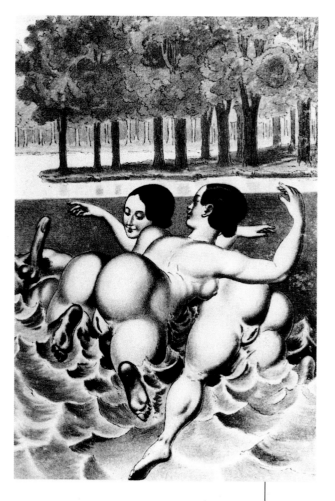

OPPOSITE PAGE: *Les Baigneuses*, August Renoir 1841-1919
TOP: Watercolour, Peter Fendi, 1796-1842

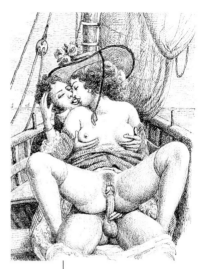

Swimming stimulates the whole of our skin surface, like some all-embracing lover. Only sex itself is more comprehensively sensual than swimming naked. All the hairs on the body move like weed in the tide, and the current is like persistent fingers exploring every part, caressing every nerve ending. Unfortunately, making love in water – although it is good fun occasionally and everyone should try it – does not combine the pleasures of swimming and sex in an orgasmic tidal wave. Indeed waves are one of the problems in the sea, together with buoyancy, a sense that the frenzied movement might provoke shark attack, and a fear not of being seen so much as rescued. Even in the safety and privacy of a swimming pool, making love in the water is no more than an erotic novelty. It is as if our bodies produce a local anaesthetic in the sex organs to prevent sensory overload. But making love before or after swimming – that is quite another thing.

Sex contains all, bodies, souls,

Meanings, proofs, purities, delicacies, results, promulgations,

Songs, commands, health, pride, the maternal mystery, the seminal milk,

All hopes, benefactions, bestowals, all the passions, loves, beauties,

                                               delights of the earth,

All the governments, judges, gods, followed persons of the earth,

These are contained in sex as parts of itself and justifications of itself.

Without shame the man I like knows and avows the deliciousness of his sex,

Without shame the woman I like knows and avows hers.

                                  Walt Whitman, 1819-1892

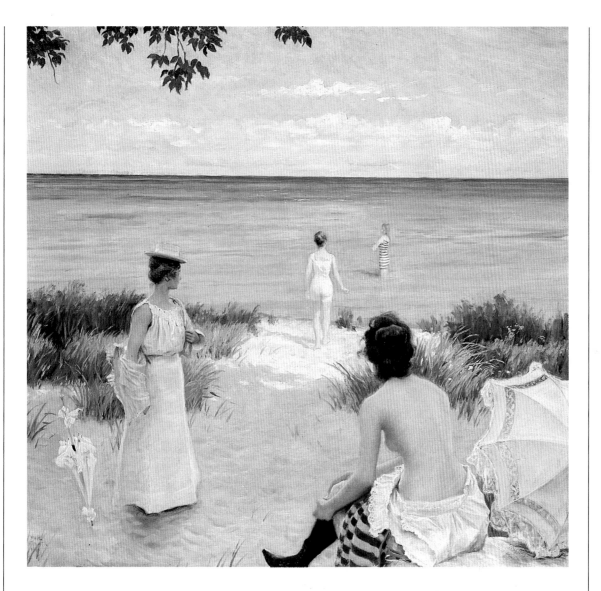

OPPOSITE PAGE: Drawing by an unknown French artist, circa 1930
ABOVE: *Bathers on Hornbaek Beach 1900*, Paul Fischer, 1860-1934

FURTHER READING

THE SENSES: There is no better general introduction to the subject than *A Natural History of The Senses* by Diane Ackerman, Random House and Chapmans 1990: lively scholarship written from a personal perspective. Also of interest: *The Sense of Smell,* Roy Bedichek, Doubleday and Michael Joseph 1960. *The Physiology of Taste,* A. Brillat Savarin (translated by M.F.K. Fisher) North Point Press, 1986. *The Sense of Sight,* John Berger, Pantheon Books, 1980. Touching: *The Human Significance of the Skin,* A. Montague, Columbia University Press, 1971. *'Sense and Sensibility'* The Century Magazine, Vol. 75, Feb.1908, Helen Keller

EROTICA: *Eros: an erotic journey through the senses* by Carlo Scipione Ferrero, Mondadori 1988 is a rich personal account. The anthologies of erotic art and literature: *Erotica* and *Erotica II,* Carroll and Graf and Littlebrown 1992 and 1993 give good general coverage. Also of interest: *The Erotic Arts,* Peter Webb, Secker and Warburg revised 1983: the standard work on the subject. *Geschichte der erotischer Kunst,* Eduard Fuchs, Munich 1908. *Eros Revived,* Peter Wagner, Secker and Warburg 1988. Although many works of erotic fiction have been made available to a wider public (notably by Grove Press in the USA and W.H.Allen in the UK) there is much that has not been reprinted. The greatest collection of this material is in the British Library, and the best guide to it is *The Private Case,* Patrick John Kearney, Jay Landesman, 1981

GENERAL: *The History of Sexuality,* Michel Foucault, Gallimard 1976, translation Random House 1978 (see also volume 2). *Intimate Behaviour,* Desmond Morris, Bantam 1973. *Studies in the Psychology of Sex,* Havelock Ellis, F.A. Davis 1928. *The Joy of Sex,* Alex Comfort, Quartet 1974. *The Illustrated Kama Sutra,* Hamlyn, 1987. *Oriental Erotic Art,* Philip Rawson, John Calmann and Cooper,1980. Most of the texts referred to and quoted can be found in standard bibliographies. Translations especially recommended are George Holden's translation of *Nana,* Penguin 1972, W.R.Trask's *Casanova, History of My Life,* Penguin and Harcourt Brace Jovanavich and Alistair Eliot's *Femmes/Hombres* of Verlaine, Anvil Press 1979.